COPYRIGHT NOTICE

Disclaimer

The content provided in this book is for informational purposes only and is not a substitute for medical advice, diagnosis or treatment.

as the days go by

A Better Life

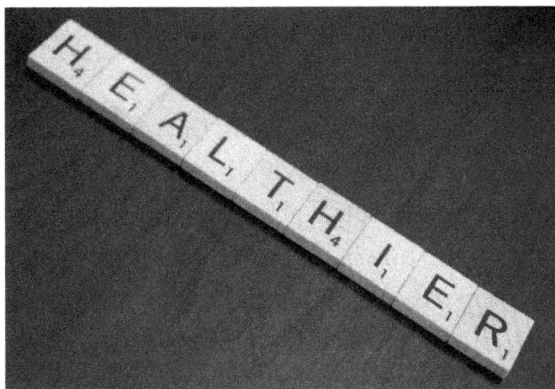

Photo Credit: Thomas Haynie.

A Letter From the Publisher.

There are those of us who have genetic disposition to certain kinds of health problems. There are those of us who live without health insurance. There are also those of us who are forced into unhealthy conditions by our families, or communities, or governments.

This is not a book to take on all the problems in the world today about health. It is a book to help all of us see what is already available, so that we can all aspire to live a better life.

In the subtitle of this book, you're told that there will be *a step-by-step guide to a healthier and happier life.*

Throughout the book you will find information about many things. The most important thing about this book is that it gives you information from diverse experts. For example, from diverse experts you find out what to eat, when to eat, and even how to eat. We think food is a big factor in a healthier living. We are what we eat. Our body is just composed of different organs working together. The more *good* fuel they have, the *better* they work. It is only common sense.

You will also see discussions on the importance of sleep, meditation, and gratitude. We all know that we still don't understand different things about our lives, about our bodies, and about our universe. The brain is one of those mysteries. For some reason, research keeps showing that sleep, meditation, and gratitude all help our psyche.

In other words, to really be healthier, we need both the right physical and psychological "foods," so to speak. If you only use the right physical stuff, your body will be good, and that is great. But, sooner or later, your psyche will catch up with you and you will end up eating badly, and go straight back to an unhealthier physical body.

So, both are important. That is why diets alone don't work. It has to be a lifestyle. It has to be something that works with both the outside and the inside.

Therefore, if you put everything we have in this book into practice, we could safely say that there will be a better you. It stars from day one, and life only gets better.

Thank you for purchasing this book, and supporting its author.

Sincerely,

011 Media Team

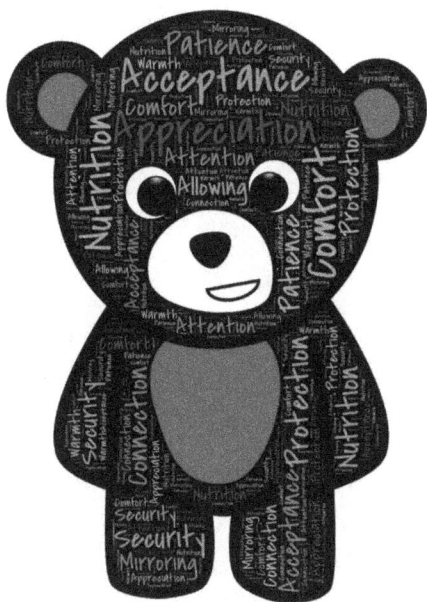

We Have Needs

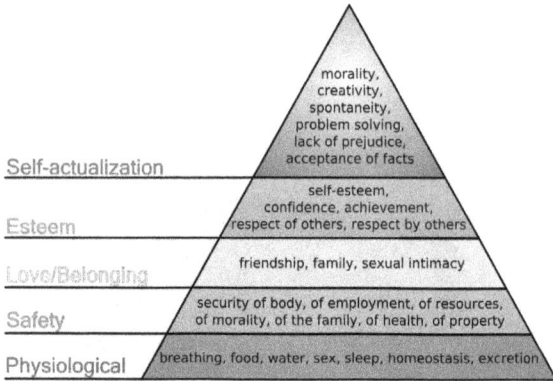

Photo Credit: J. Finkelstein.

Humans have needs; you already know that because you're human. You eat, you drink, you sleep, and you want happiness.

According to Abraham Maslow, who was an American psychologist that influenced our understanding of personality, there are needs that are much deeper than basic needs, which a person needs to satisfy in order to live a happy life.

He created a pyramid out of these needs. They go from lower needs, which include basic needs such as eating or sex, to higher needs, which include advanced needs such as morality or creativity. In between these, you have middle needs, which include things like friendship and self-esteem.

What is interesting about his theory is that it is based on two inter-dependent beliefs: that one need or another constantly motived the whole person; and that the person needed to satisfy lower needs in order to reach higher needs.

What this says is that if you're starving yourself through crazy diets, or you don't fulfill your sexual needs, don't expect to reach enlightenment and encounter the elusive happiness because it could be the case that you're abandoning that one need that may be motivating everything.

Yeah, stops you in your tracks, doesn't it?

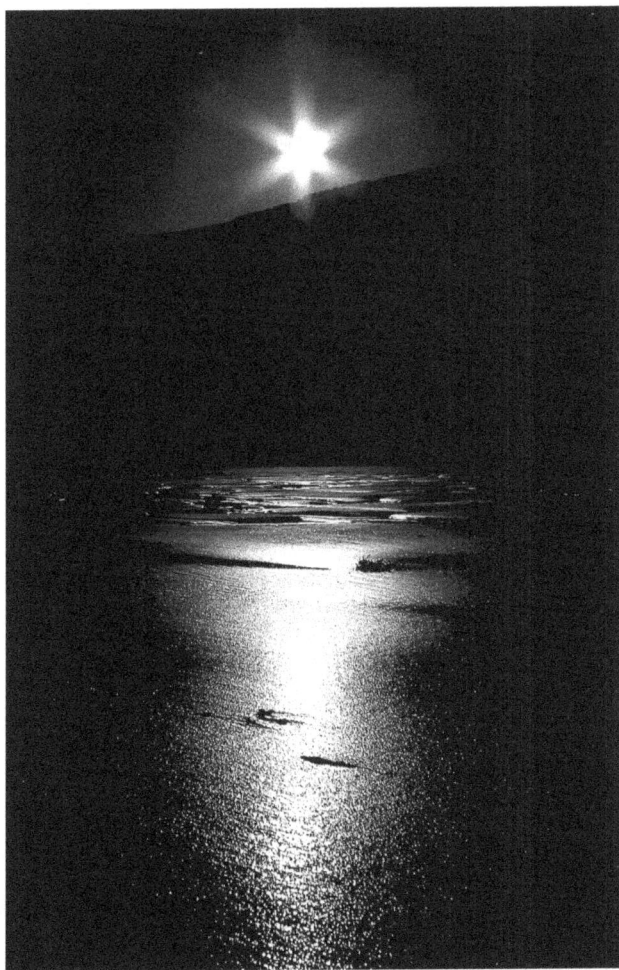

Tonight Is The Night

Start tonight. No, really, starting is best at night. Why? Because your body will wake up the next day, and it will be ready for all the challenges ahead.

Have you heard the expression, "Everyday is a new day"? Well, it couldn't be any truer in this case.

So, it starts tonight.

But before we start your night, we need to make sure you and your bedroom are ready for the night.

Let's go!

Feng Shui

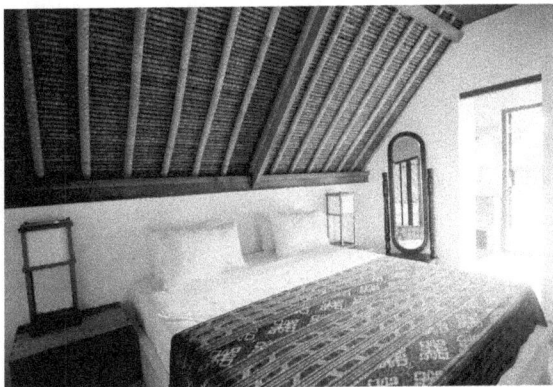

Photo Credit: Bart Speelman.

You have heard it everywhere. It is just one of those phrases that keeps popping up wherever you go, and you hear it on television and even radio, yet many of us have no idea what it is all about.

Feng shui, which translates to "wind water" in Mandarin, is a Chinese philosophical system that dates back to five thousand years. It is a system that seeks to harmonize human life with the environment.

Of course, one of the most important environmental surroundings is our home. The bedroom is an important room to feng shui, according to Cathy Wong, a licensed naturopathic doctor who writes for the popular website *About.com*, because it affects the quality of our sleep.

How do you feng shui your bedroom? One important way is to make sure the bed is not facing the window or the door. This gives you a sense of safety, which aids you to sleep better.

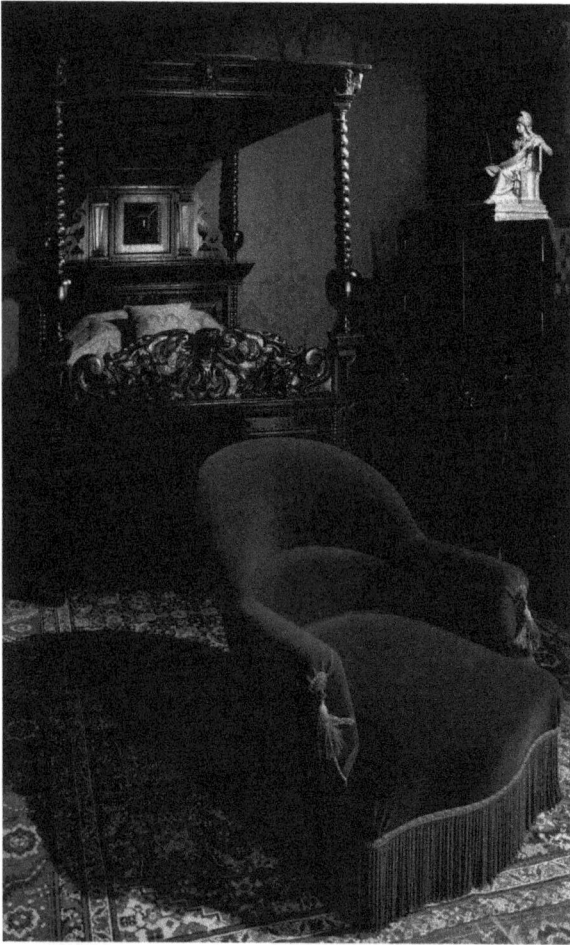

Jayme Barrett, author of *Feng Shui Your Life*, suggests keeping the items in the bedroom in twos as that creates harmony. This is rooted in the Chinese philosophy of ying and yang.

According to Casey Kochmer, the author of *A Personal Tao*, ying and yang are two halves that make up one wholesome. But the point of the ying and yang is not to say it is absolute because "when you split something into two halves," argues Kochmer, "it upsets the equilibrium of wholeness. This starts both halves chasing after each other as they seek a new balance with each other."

In other words, by having things in twos you're seeking wholesomeness for your bedroom. Another important way to keep your bedroom personal is to display things that are just for you.

HGTV's Leah Hennen recommends choosing artworks that depicts things you want to manifest in life. You want to go to an interesting destination? Perhaps a painting of Trinidad! You're thinking of getting pregnant? Perhaps a painting of ... Well, you get the idea.

Although there are many other ways to feng shui your bedrooms, as well as your home in general, these simple and easy to follow recommendations will get you off to a good start.

Color

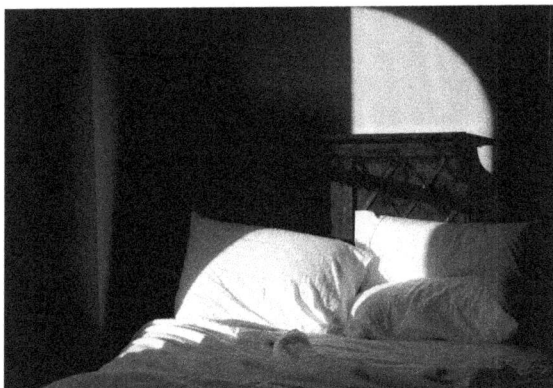

Photo Credit: Lillian Nelson.

Color. Do you cringe when you hear that? I did not like color. In fact, you could say I was very much afraid of it. However, science has proven time and again that color is good for us.

According to Rebecca Soskin, an interior decorator in New York City, some colors can make you pretty relaxed. If you know what hues to pick, she says, it can help you to unwind.

So what colors should you choose? Travelodge surveyed 2,000 guests at their hotels and found that those whose bedroom walls were colored blue slept the longest, while purple walls led to the least amount of sleep.

What is the big deal about blue? Psychological studies have been done on color and they found that blue is a color that calms the mind and body, lowers blood pressure and heart rate, and decreases unwanted feelings like anxiety and aggression.

One way to get blue into your bedroom is to find an image you like.

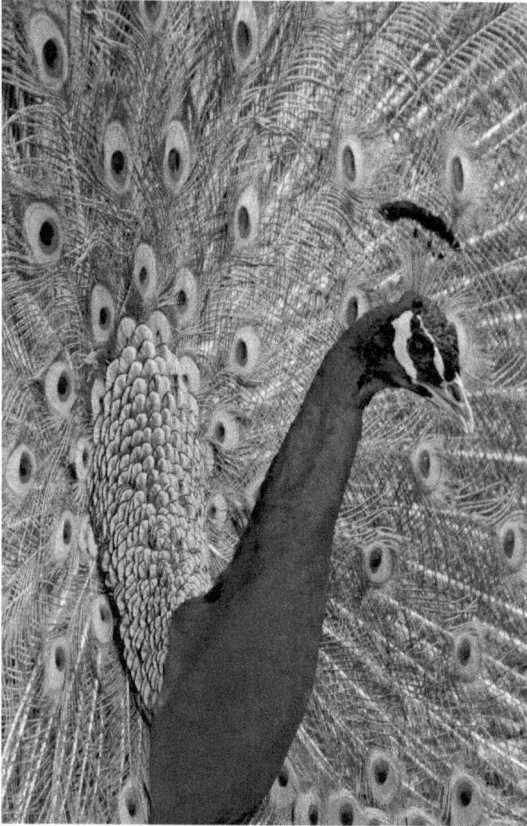

If blue is not your favorite color, try yellow and green. They ranked high in the Travelodge survey, while grey and brown ranked lowest.

Senses

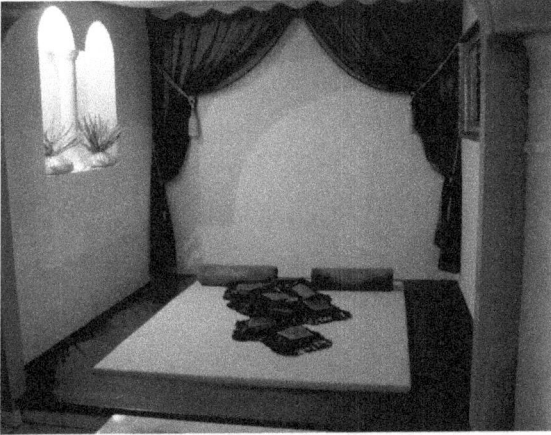

Photo Credit: Enrico Corno.

Did you know that what you see, hear, smell, taste, or touch in your bedroom can affect your sleep? The Sleep Foundation did an entire project on the bedroom, and one of their main education focuses is on this. See if your bedroom can be upgraded as far as the senses are concerned:

Light; What you see is probably the most important. If you're seeing light, whether natural or unnatural, it is going to tell your brain that it is not yet the time to sleep.

If you didn't have electricity or electronic products in your home, your body would start to feel sleepy after dark.

If you're watching dramatic television then that light is going right to your brain, and your brain thinks it is still light out.

So tune out the light, darken your room, and try to give yourself time to adjust to it by slowly fading out the different lights you're exposed to. For example, if you turn off some of your lights in your home, and then turn off your cell phone, and then turn off the television, et cetera.

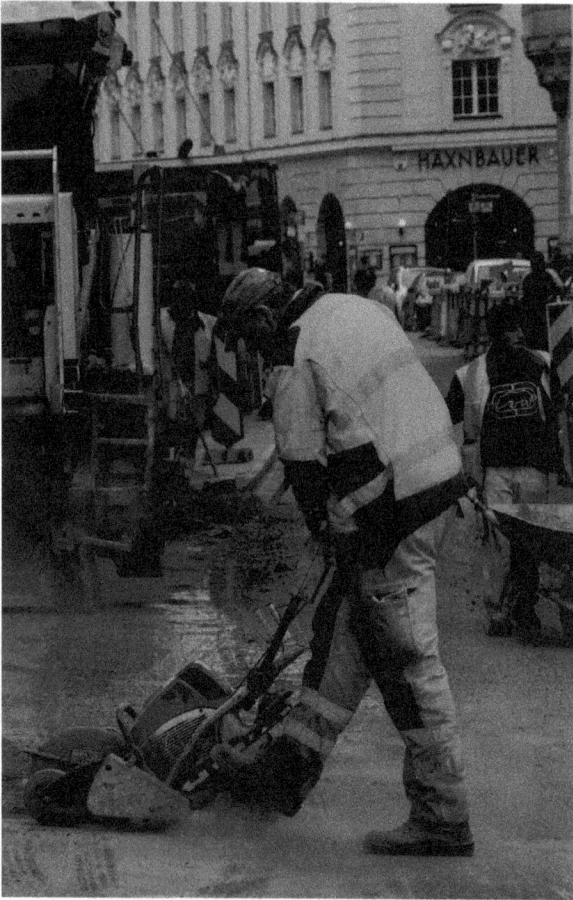

Sound; If you're hearing the fire trucks going down in your main street, the cars passing by near your window, or bars blasting music in the neighborhood, chances are you're probably not going to have a good night's sleep.

Ever hear the expression, "Fire with fire"? In this case it actually works. So, you tune out the noise with noise! White noise, as it is called, is a type of noise that helps the brain to get distracted from the actual noise pollution we are met with in our environment and helps us to sleep better.

Psychiatrist David Neubauer, who also happens to be the director of the Johns Hopkins Sleep Disorders Center, says white noise is very soothing.

White noise is good because it is steady, and therefore is not interrupting your sleep; and yet it works as a distraction from other noises.

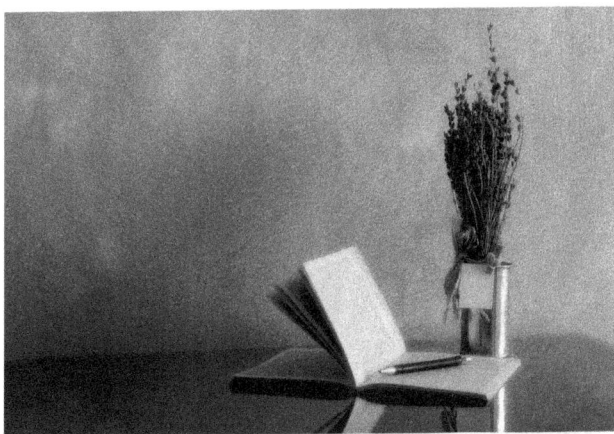

Smell; What you smell as you sleep is another factor in whether you do or do not get the good rest you need.

What type of scents help with sleep? Lavender, for example. Tiffany Field, a scientist with the University of Miami School of Medicine, told *NBC News* that lavender has been shown to put people in a parasympathetic or relaxed state.

Allergies, on the other hand, are not good for sleep, says the Sleep Foundation, because sneezing can wake you up. You might not even realize it, as you may not even remember having had sneezed during the night, but it can and does. So, better to get on top of that. If you're allergic to dust, keep your bedroom as dust-free as possible.

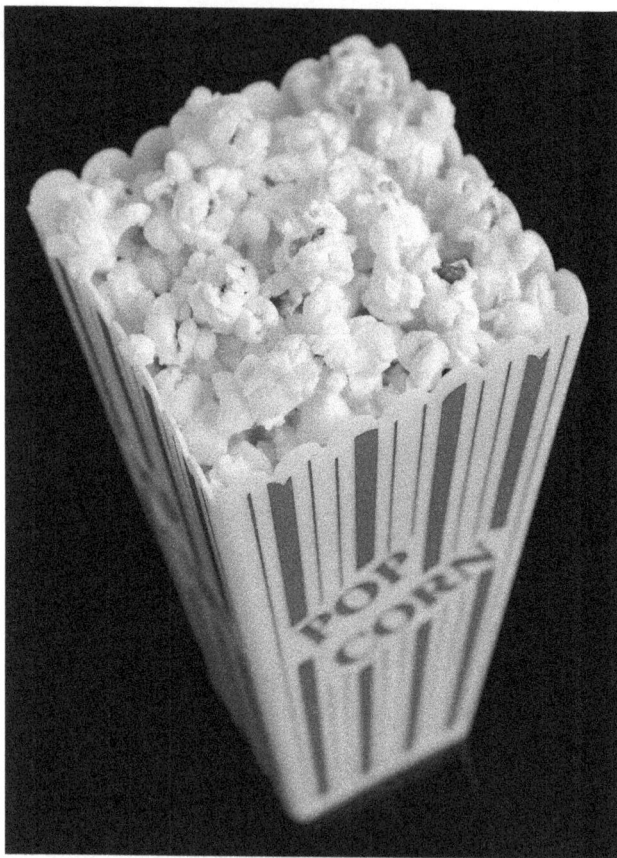

Taste; If you're in bed watching television and having your snacks, or you went to a late night movie at the local theater and had tons of popcorn, you're probably not going to have a good night's sleep.

August McLaughlin, a certified nutritionist in Los Angeles, says eating too much too close to bedtime can lead to insomnia. Similarly, she warns, going to bed too hungry will do the same.

So, what do you do? Eat your meal three hours before bed, and then have a small snack. McLaughlin recommends something like cereal and milk.

Touch; Your body, as it sleeps at night, will touch your clothes, the sheets, and the bed. So, of course, it only makes sense to make sure those things are in alignment with your body. Otherwise, you might end up not having a good night's sleep.

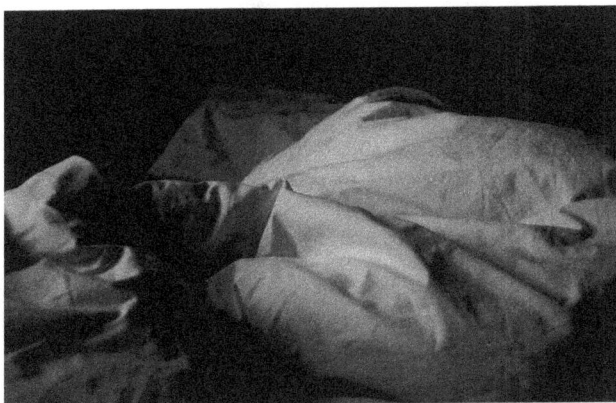

Michael Breus, a senior vice president at Phoenix Sleep, says you can release up to a half gallon of sweat and oils in one night of sleep.

What does that mean? You should have sheets that are made of natural fibers, like cotton, because they are more absorbent than synthetics.

As far as mattresses and pillows go, it really all depends on whether you're a back, side, or tummy sleeper. After all, it is just all about the comfort.

Clete Kushida, the director of the Stanford University Center for Human Sleep Research, told *CNN* that mattresses don't work miracle and that their contribution is about them being a surface that doesn't cause pain to muscles.

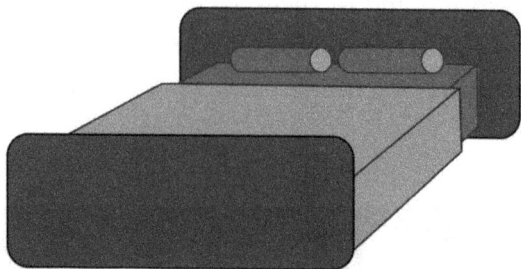

In other words a mattress has a specific purpose. Yes, there are companies out there trying o make mattresses into what they are not meant to be, just to make a buck, but in reality mattresses are just meant to keep you comfortable. Therefore, when you shop for a new mattress buy a mattress that fits with your needs... not because it can do all sorts of other tricks.

Body Clock

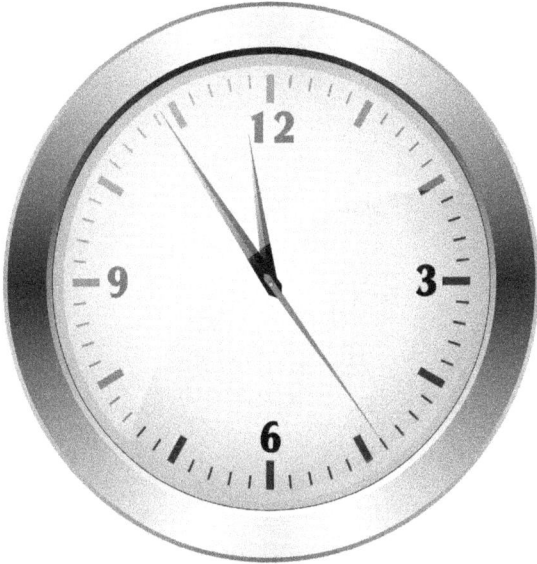

Photo Credit: Robert Proksa.

The circadian rhythm, or the body clock as it is better known, is our innate way of knowing when to wake up, when to eat, when to sleep, etc. It is a 24-hour physiological process of all living beings.

When it comes to sleep, it is important to understand that there are many factors that contribute to our success or failure in attaining a good night's sleep. However, there are two specific things that greatly influence our sleep:

Melatonin; Melatonin is a hormone produced by our bodies, which tell our bodies when to wake up and when to sleep.

According to the Mayo Clinic, melatonin is produced by the pineal gland in the brain. However, it can also be produced by some foods, although in small amounts.

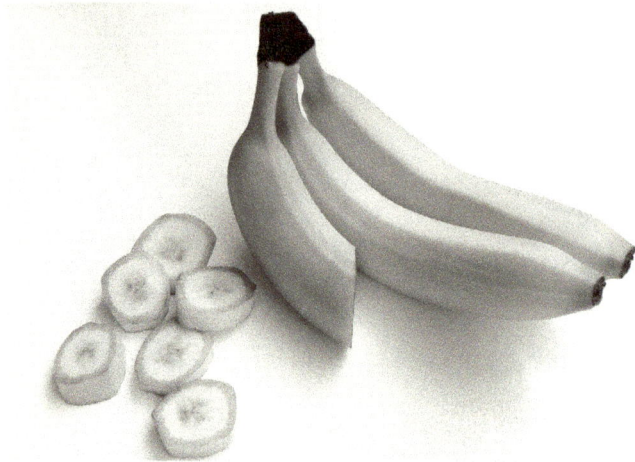

The Institute of Health Sciences says these foods, which naturally contain melatonin, include bananas, tomatoes, and radishes, as well as porridge oats, sweet corn, and even red wine.

There are also melatonin supplements for certain individuals. For example, WebMD notes that people who are may use this supplement include travelers dealing with jetlag, people who work changing shifts, and the blind who need it to establish day and night cycles.

The Sun; The sun is the source of energy for all organisms. Like all other organisms, it affects human life. The sun sends light to our cell bodies and tells them to wake us. When the sun goes down, those cells understand it is time to sleep.

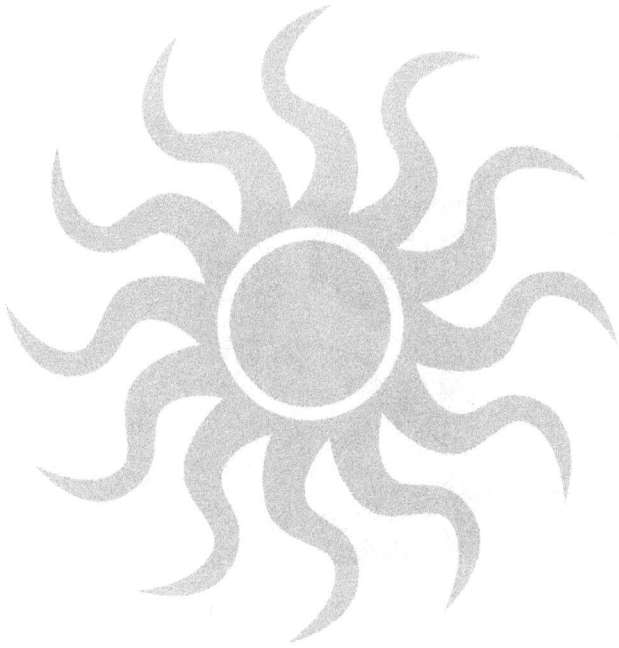

Humans have been too smart for their own good because when the sun goes down we still want more light. That is where the creation of light using incandescent, fluorescent, and/or other man-made light source came into the equation.

The International Dark-Sky Association says that not only does artificial light affect our sleep negatively but that it also increases risk for obesity, diabetes, and cancer, among other nasty things.

Of course, artificial light is useful at certain times, and it is healthy for certain individuals.

The Mayo Clinic says because the sun affects our melatonin, an individual might end up with a seasonal affective disorder or SAD during the winter months when the days are shorter.

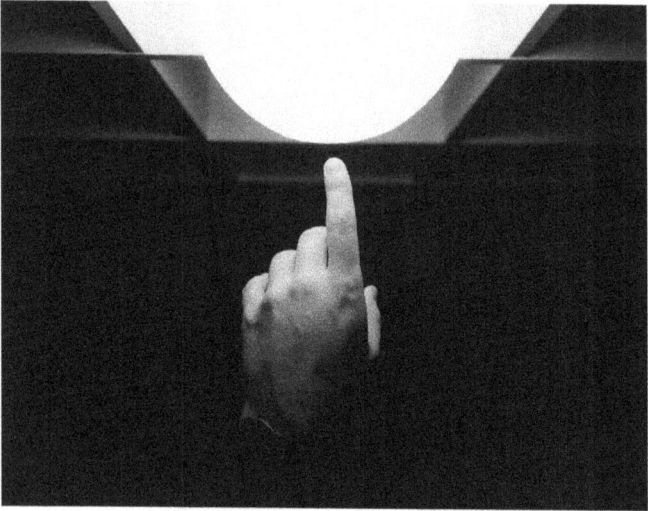

Individuals living with SAD are often prescribed sitting in front or under strong light. By doing so, their chemistry balances and their mood might positively elevate.

Water

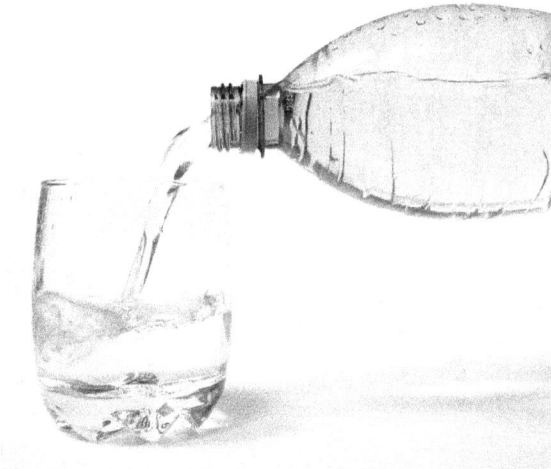

Photo Credit: Zsuzsanna Kilian.

Water is, well, very important. After all, most of your body is composed of water.

In terms of preparation for bed, you want to place a glass of water next to your bed for two reasons.

<u>Overnight</u>: While you sleep, sometimes your might snore and wake up with a dry throat. Other times you might have your saliva going down the wrong pipe, forcing you to wake up with a cough.

This could be in the middle of the nigh, and if you have to get up and go to the kitchen, chances are you might have a hard time to get back in bed.

So, it is good to have a cup of water nearby.

<u>Morning</u>: The second need is for the next morning. As

you will see in the water section, water is the first thing you will drink in the morning.

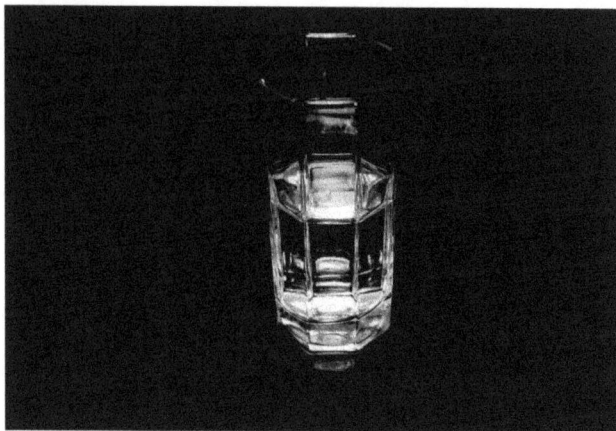

It just makes everything work better.

Best Time to Sleep

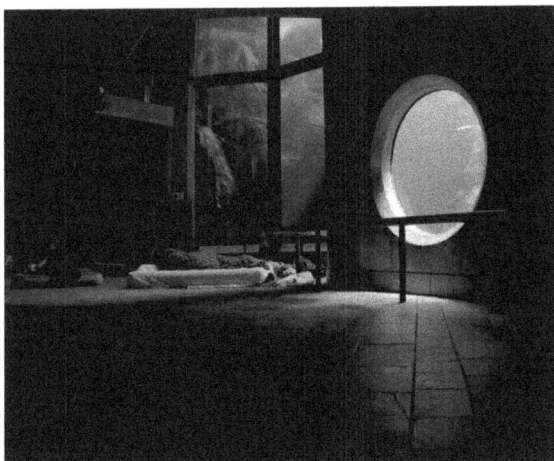

Photo Credit: Erik Charlton.

Yeah, sleep! You might be thinking to yourself, "Why is this person telling me to sleep!" Well, only you can determine your sleep time.

Psychologist Michael J. Breus, the author of *Good Night: The Sleep Doctor's 4-Week Program to Better Sleep and Better Health*, everyone can figure out their perfect bedtime by adjusting their preferred wake-up time to the time they go to bed.

For example, if you're someone who wants to follow this program, you're encouraged to wake up at 6am. So, if you want to wake up at 6am, you would want to go to bed at 10:45pm.

How did Breus come up with that math? He says the average person needs five 90-minute cycles of sleep per night.

If you don't know what these cycles are, each of them is composed of what is called the five stages of sleep.

According to Kendra Cherry, a guide for the website About.com, these stages are divided into two categories of sleep known as non-rapid eye movement or Non-REM and rapid eye movement or REM.

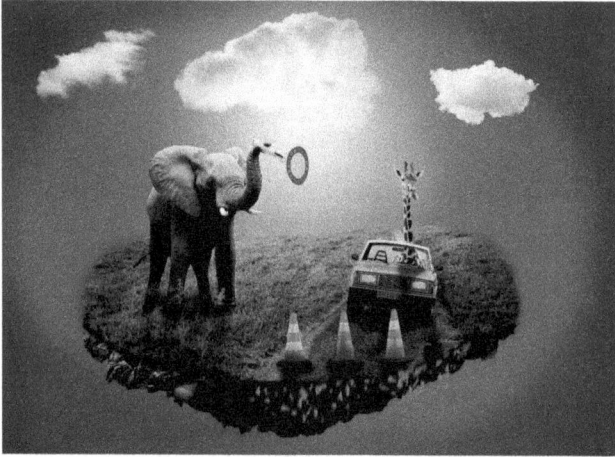

When you dream, especially when you dream surreal things, you are in stage five.

"Dreaming occurs because of increased brain activity, but voluntary muscles become paralyzed," wrote Diana L. Walcutt, a licensed psychologist in Maryland, for the popular psychological website PsychCentral.

Because our bodies are so interlinked with the sun, it is best to make sure we wake up around sunrise. So, wherever you are in the world you can use the 7.5 hours before that to work into your sleep.

However, Breus points out that not everyone sleeps 7.5, different people might need different amounts of sleep.

Water Is Our Friend

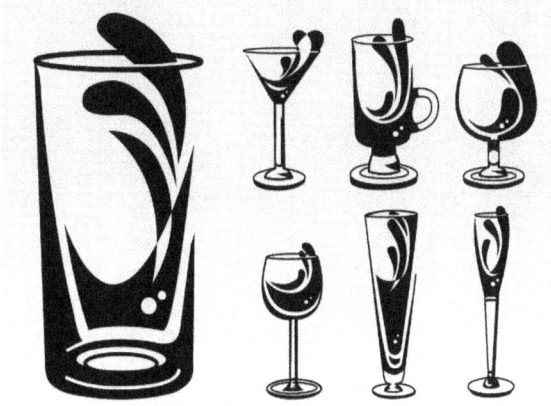

Photo Credit: Kimberly Vohsen.

Did you like drinking plain water as a child? I didn't. In fact, I remember getting nauseous at the sight of it. It just tasted nothing; it had nothing to offer other than what mom told me about it.

According to Mayo Clinic, however, water is the most important thing in your life. That is because water is the "principal chemical component and makes up about 60 percent of your body weight. Every system in your body depends on water."

So, let's understand the relationship between water and our bodies better.

Start Drinking Early

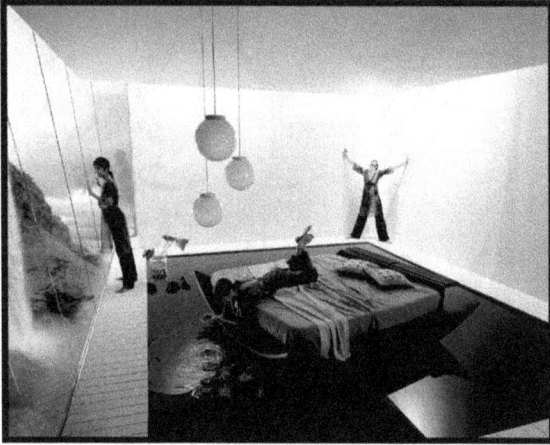

Photo Credit: Mazzali Armadi

What do you do the first thing when you wake up? If you are like millions of people worldwide, you probably have a cup of tea or coffee. You want to jump start your life.

But that is not the way to go.

According to Dr. Adam Dave, a regular on the Livestrong Foundation's livestrong.org website and the author of *The Paradigm Diet*, while "drinking water at any time is beneficial to your health, consuming a big glass first thing in the morning brings unique rewards."

Dave is not the only one who feels this way. Dr. Akilah El, who is based in both Atlanta and Munich, says that water in the morning is the best thing, especially if you can add lemon.

El says the combination provides many health benefits

such as preventing allergies and infections, strengthening the liver functions, and aiding in weight loss.

Basically, it is just better to start drinking early. After reading the next part, you will understand why.

Lots of Water

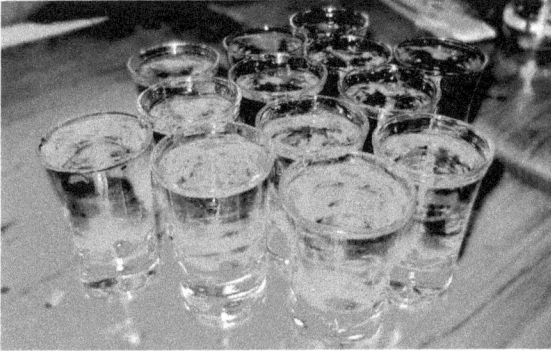

Photo Credit: Frédéric Dupont.

Now that you understand the importance of water, the natural question to ask is how much of it do you really need?

That depends.

For children, generally it depends on their age. According to Ashima Kant and Barry Graubard, researchers at Queens College in New York, five to eight glasses a day are good.

When it comes to the adults, however, most people are duped by that "eight glasses a day" myth. According to the Institute of Medicine, which is under the National Academy of Sciences, a healthy adult woman needs about 91 ounces while a healthy adult man would need about 125 ounces per day.

That means, for a healthy adult woman about 11 cups of water; and while a healthy adult man would be looking at

16 cups!

Now you understand why starting early in the morning will be a big help!

As you go through your day those cups get out of the way if you plan them right. After waking up, during your exercise, after exercise, with your breakfast, with your lunch, with your dinner, et cetera, and you will see those cups disappear.

Types of Water

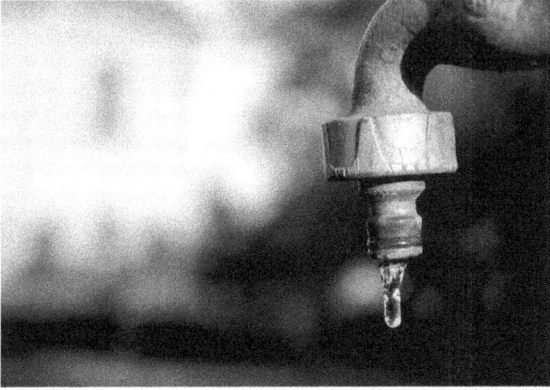

Photo Credit: Mateusz Stachowski.

Did you know that tap water is pretty good? No, I didn't know that. Like many of you, I depended on bottled water for my drinking.

According to an article by webmd.com reviewed by Dr. Brunilda Nazario, a doctor certified in both Florida and Gerogia, There are many cities with clean water. New York City, for example, has some of the purest and safest drinking water in the world.

That, of course, does not mean all water coming out of the tap is created equal. Every city is different, every home is different.

The Environmental Protection Agency (EPA) works hard to make sure water is safe, and the local water organizations can go above and beyond the safe limits, but at the end of the day it all has to do with you, where you live, and what type of system you're using.

For example, if you live in a building whose water pipes are really old and rusty, chances are your water may not be so pure and safe.

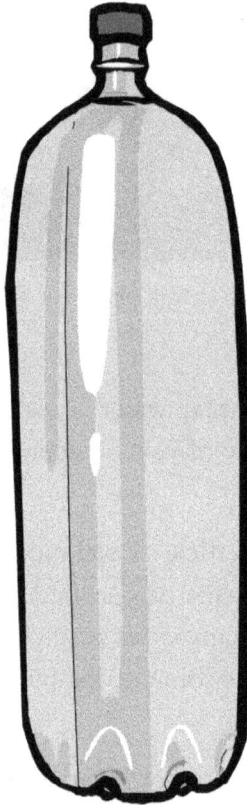

But what about bottled water?

It is important to understand first that bottled water and tap water are managed differently. The Mayo Clinic says that the Food and Drug Administration (FDA) oversees bottled water, while the EPA regulates generic water.

In 2005, the ABC show *20/20* ran a segment on the issue of bottled water versus tap water.

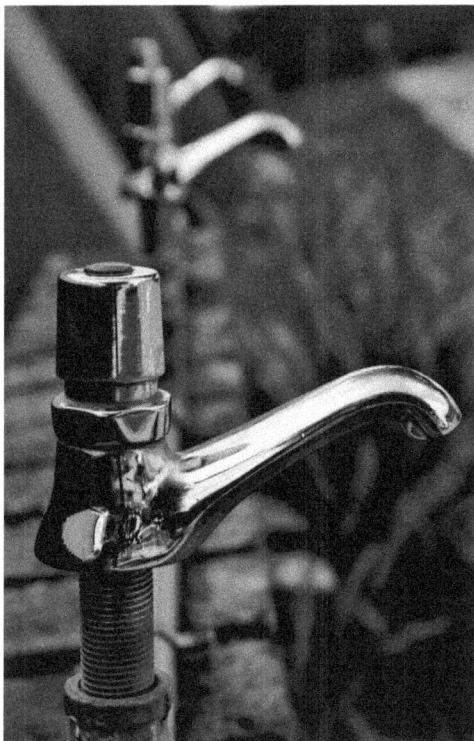

They took samples from five of the popular bottled water brands and samples from New York City tap water, and they sent them to a lab at the University of New Hampshire. What did they find? The evaluation found no difference between the two types of water.

That said, Mayo Clinic does note the fact that some individuals have vulnerability to contaminants that may be found in regular water. These individuals include people living with HIV/AIDS, those undergoing chemotherapy, as well as those who have received a transplant.

What other sources are there for water?

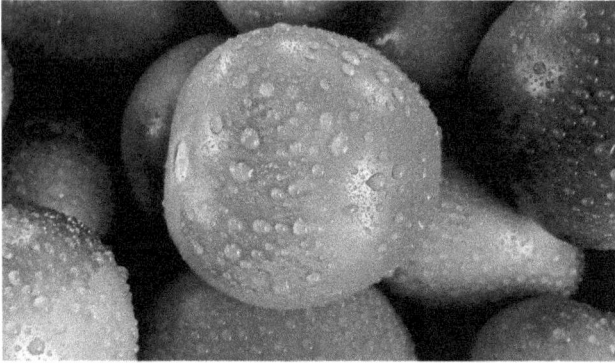

How about food! Yes, the Institute on Medicine estimates about 20% of our water comes from food.

Dr. Howard Murad, a professor of medicine at UCLA and the author of *The Water Secret*, it is just as important to eat foods that help you to stay hydrated.

In his book, Murad has chapter called "eat your water," in which he talks about how certain foods help us to retain our water longer.

What type of foods? Murad says to replace "at least one glass of water a day with one serving of raw fruits or vegetables to stay hydrated significantly longer."

Foods that allow this include greens and vegetables like broccoli and avocado, and fruits like mango and pomegranate.

Finally, there is something to keep in mind. Drinking

too much water *can* kill you. Yes, you read that correctly.

It has happened. In most of these cases, it had to do with drinking large quantities of water in short time. For example, a woman in Brazil was a contestant on a radio show and drank over a gallon of water within an hour, leaving her to collapse and die from a stroke.

So, if you are going outside the limits set by the Institute of Medicine, talk to your doctor first and see if that is a good idea for you.

Being Actively Alive

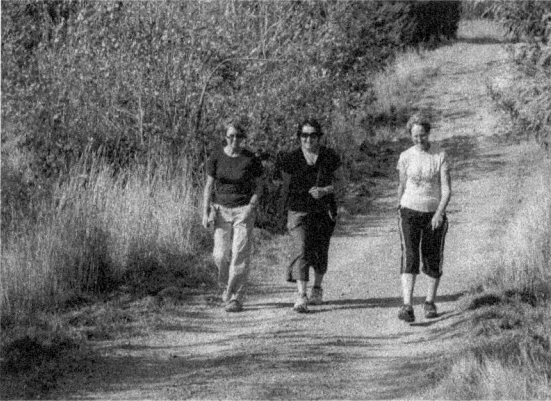

Photo Credit: Phil Norton.

When some of us hear the word "exercise" we cringe, because we immediately imagine the machines at the gym. The word just means to engage in physical activity to sustain or improve health.

The ladies you see in Phil Norton's image up there, they are hiking, one of the many types of physical activity at our disposal. The image is a powerful reminder of how nature can be a good source of support if you let it.

If you look at the image, what do you see? What do you think these women are doing? What do you think they are talking about?

They might be gossiping, or enjoying a good laugh about something that has happened to one of them, or it could be the case they are just in a good mood because they are hanging out with each other.

According to Jen Lasky of *Everyday Health*, hiking is a surprising way to burn calories because, by just moving moderately on a nice scenic walk with a friend or two, you can end up burning about 200 calories.

But is exercise all about calories? Is hiking the only way to get exercise?

No, of course, not.

Benefits of Exercise

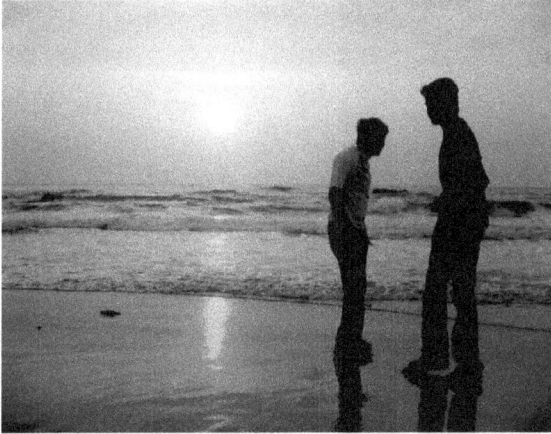

Photo Credit: Barun Patro.

We have all heard it that exercise is good for us. Our families, our friends, our health professionals, even our government tells us so. But how exactly is it good for us, and what are the benefits?

Physical activity has many benefits to our well being. It helps us to feel better, gives us more energy, and will even help us to live longer.

Mayo Clinic put together seven of the best benefits physical activity ultimately gives us:

1) **Controls weight** through prevention of excess weight, or maintaining weight loss.

This is a benefit that is known to most of us, and it is probably what we think about when we think about physical activity. It is what others see, and it is what many of us are motivated by.

2) **Prevents, manages, or even improves health problems** like heart disease, diabetes, some cancers, arthritis, depression, and a bunch of other health problems. I would say this is really an important thing to keep in mind about physical activity.

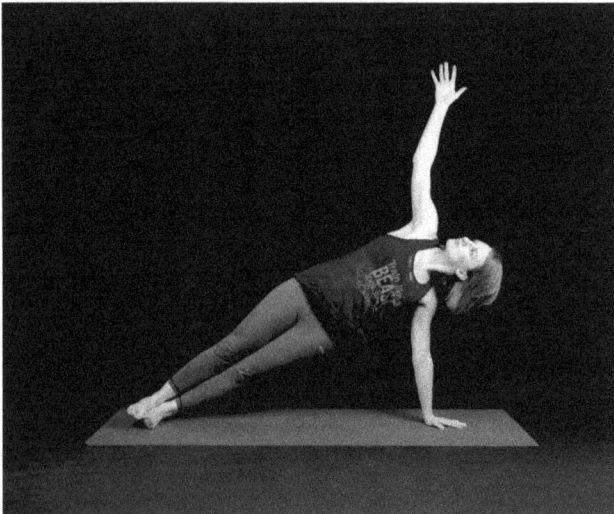

3) **Improves mood** by stimulating brain chemicals that deal with feeling confident, self-esteem, happiness, and relaxation. In other words physical activity can keep us sane, or at least balancing our moods.

4) **Boosts energy** by strengthening muscles, engaging endurance, and delivering oxygen to the heart and lungs.

5) **Promotes better sleep** by helping with falling asleep, as well as deepening the sleep, so long as it is not too

close to bedtime.

6) **Promotes better sex life** by leading to an enhanced arousal for women and by helping prevent erectile dysfunction for men.

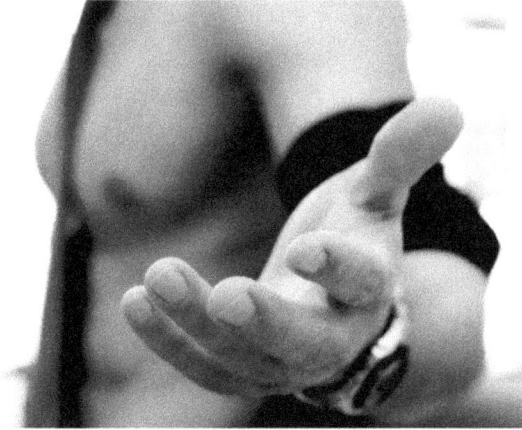

Well, this will get everyone motivated.

7) **Promotes better social life** by helping us to connect with others such as family and friends through social activities.

These benefits are tangible benefits. They are not myths or unsubstantiated ideas.

But, what type of physical activities?

Types of Exercises

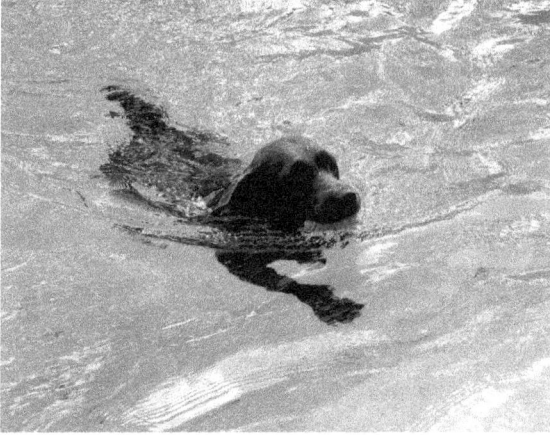

Photo Credit: Esteban Lussich.

There are many types of exercise just like there are many types of personalities. It really all depends on what you may like, or what you may consider is best for your life.

That said; let's ask the professionals. *HEALTHbeat*, which is a publication of the Harvard Medical School, pointed out five of the best ways to exercises:

1) **Swimming** is placed at the top because it has very little impact on the joints because the water supports the body, and because research has proven that it improves mental state.

Swimming forces you to use several muscle groups. Look at that dog, having to keep head up while moving legs and arms. In other words the dog is getting physical activity on at least three muscle groups!

2) **Tai Chi** is another great form of exercise because it is good for both body and mine as it incorporates movements and relaxation at the same time.

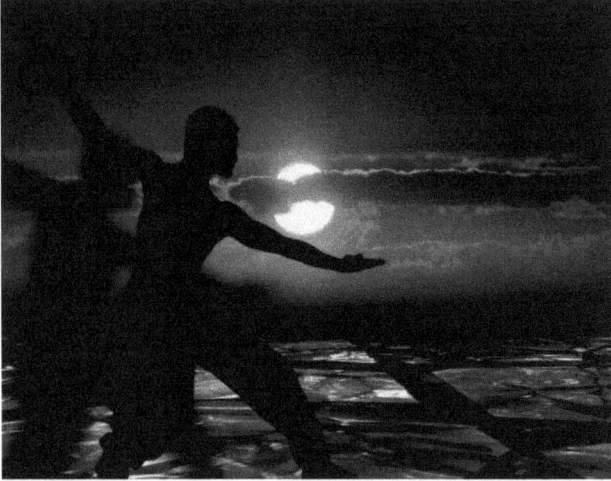

Tai Chi is rooted in Chinese culture where it was used as both defense training and internal well being. Today you can find Tai Chi groups all over the country, as it is almost as popular as yoga.

3) **Strength training** strengthens the muscles, which burn calories on their own at resting level and makes it easier to maintain a healthy weight.

4) **Walking** is positive on all levels because it can help with improving cholesterol levels, strengthens the bones, keeps the blood pressure in check, lifts mood and lowers the risks for various diseases.

5) **Kegel exercises** are important because they prevent

incontinence, and are good for both men and women, although women might be more familiar with them.

These exercises might seem like easy to do, but they require commitment to be successful. Now that you know the best exercises, the natural question to follow is: when is the best time to exercise?

Best Time to Exercise

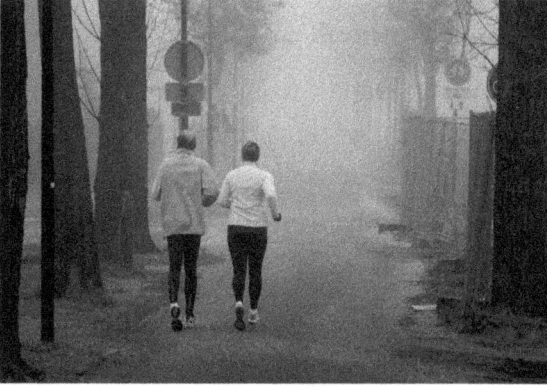

Photo Credit: Patrick Nijhuis.

The best time to exercise, again, depends on you. There are people who like to exercise in the morning, afternoon, or early evening. It depends on many things, such as when they feel like they can commit more to an activity.

Similarly, different professionals recommend different times. According to a research led by Emma Stevenson, a Senior Lecturer in Sport and Exercise Nutrition at Northumbria University in the United Kingdom, the best time to exercise is before breakfast.

Stevenson's research, which was published in the *British Journal of Nutrition*, showed that people who exercised before breakfast had burned 20% more calories than those who exercised after breakfast.

How is this possible?

"When you exercise (after fasting), your adrenaline is high and your insulin is low," Peter Hespel, a professor of exercise physiology at the University of Leuven in Belgium, told the *Associated Press*. "That ratio is favorable for your muscles to oxidize (break down) more fatty acids."

This is very different from research in the past, which recommended not working out on an empty stomach. However, it should be noted that almost all professionals have always recommended not working out within 30-45 minutes after eating.

We Are What We Eat

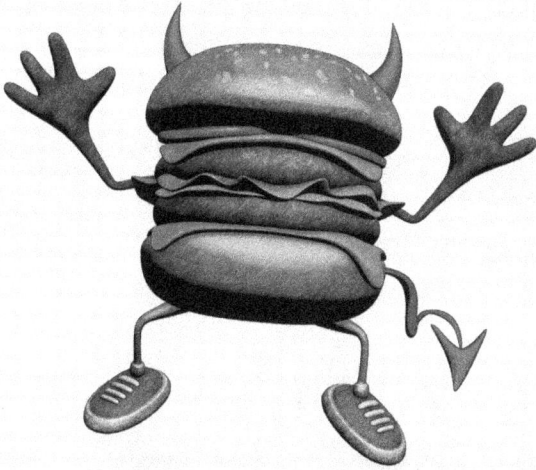

Photo Credit: Julien Tromeur.

Did you ever notice the evolutionary of our foods, as our bodies grow from being a child and into adult? Remember how what tasted awful at one stage of development ended up becoming delicious at another?

Spinach, for example, used to make me want throw up as a child. I thought it was gross, and I did not like the feeling of it in my mouth--that slimy, gooey feel.

Today, however, I love spinach! Anything that has spinach in it, I love. I could think of many other foods for which my taste had evolved in time.

Of course, it is also the opposite. Remember your delight in fast food and soda? Now, as an adult, you probably feel a tad bit guilty when you indulge in them. I sure do!

Well, guess what, the same thing happens with our culture of food as a society, too. For example, according to Katy Steinmetz of *Time* magazine, in the early 20th Century around 50% of Americans were farmers.

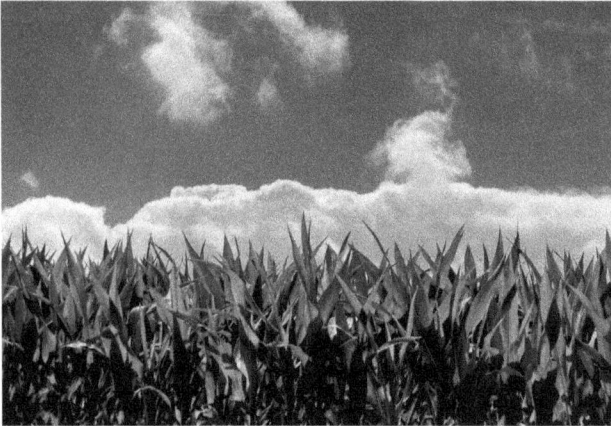

Today, according to the American Farm Bureau Federation, around 2% of Americans are farmers. It is because the industrial age had managed to create far more than before.

The same thing is also true for particular foods with particular groups within the society. According to Donna R. Gabaccia, author of *We Are What We Eat*, bagels used to be only eaten by Jews in the 1890s America, as it was only something Jews from Eastern Europe knew or liked.

Today, bagels are as American as anything else. In her book, Gabaccia writes about a Pakistani-American who sells New York style bagels in Houston in the 1990s and whose customers were neither Jewish nor New Yorkers.

So, what exactly is, or should be, the American diet?

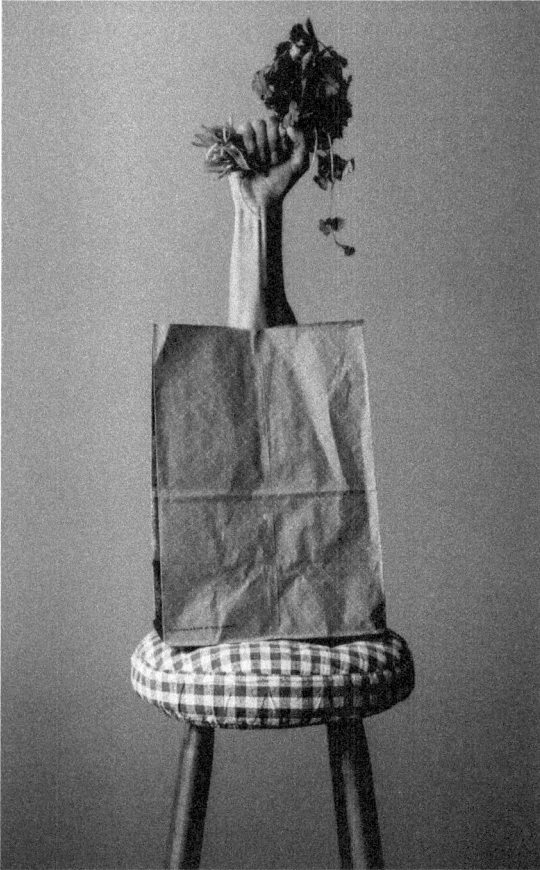

Back in 2011, the Department of Health and Human Services released its *Dietary Guidelines for Americans, 2010*, emphasizing on 3 major goals for the country: balance calories with physical activity to manage weight; consume more of certain foods and nutrients such as fruits, vegetables, whole grains, fat-free and low-fat dairy products, and seafood; and consume fewer foods with sodium (salt), saturated fats, trans fats, cholesterol, added sugars, and refined grains.

So, throughout this book I will tackle the issue of what to eat for a better health.

Red and Processed Meats

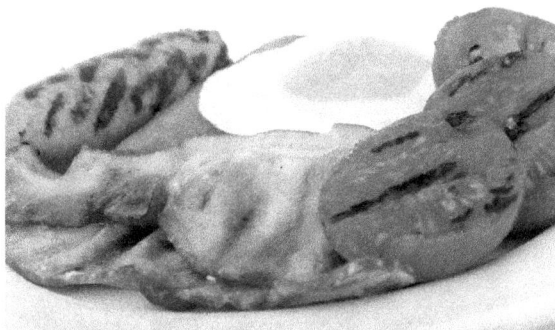

Photo Credit: JCB Spares.

If you're going to eat meat, which I'm not a big fan of, then try to at least limit your red and processed meats.

The good folks at WebMD discussed a report from the World Cancer Research Fund and the American Institute for Cancer Research, which said that said that there is a convincing evidence "for a link between red meat, processed meat, and colorectal cancer, and limited but suggestive for links to lung, esophageal, stomach, pancreatic, and endometrial cancers."

Are there some studies that say red and processed meats are perfectly fine? Of course, there are. But they are in the minority.

"The level of evidence is what people look at," Rashmi Sinha, PhD, the lead author of the National Cancer Institute study, told WebMD. "If there are 20 studies that say one thing and two studies that say the other thing, you believe the 20 studies."

Why are red and processed meats so risky? The answer could be that they come with high numbers of the wrong things.

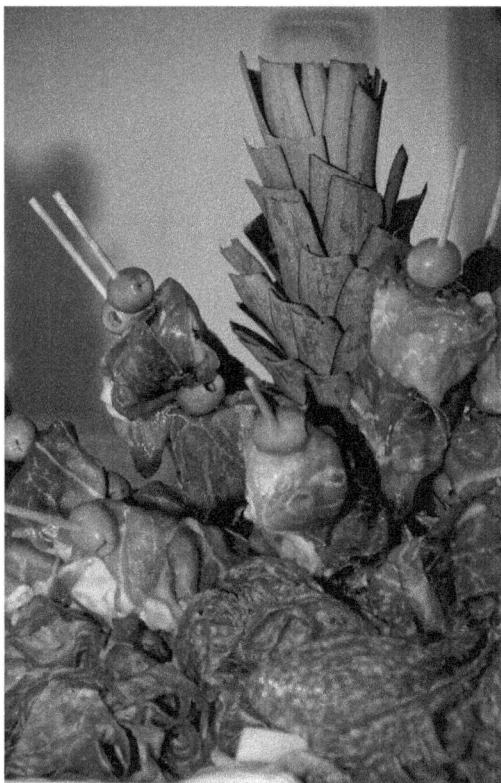

"Bacon and sausages have around 16 times more saturated fat per gram than tofu," notes Michael Mosley, a medical doctor who did an investigation behind the headlines for BBC's science and documentary series, *Horizon*.

Mosley also explained what red and processed meats

are. He said that red meats include beef, lamb, and pork; while processed meats include salami, ham, and sausages.

It is not just about cancer, red and processed meats pose higher risks for different health issues.

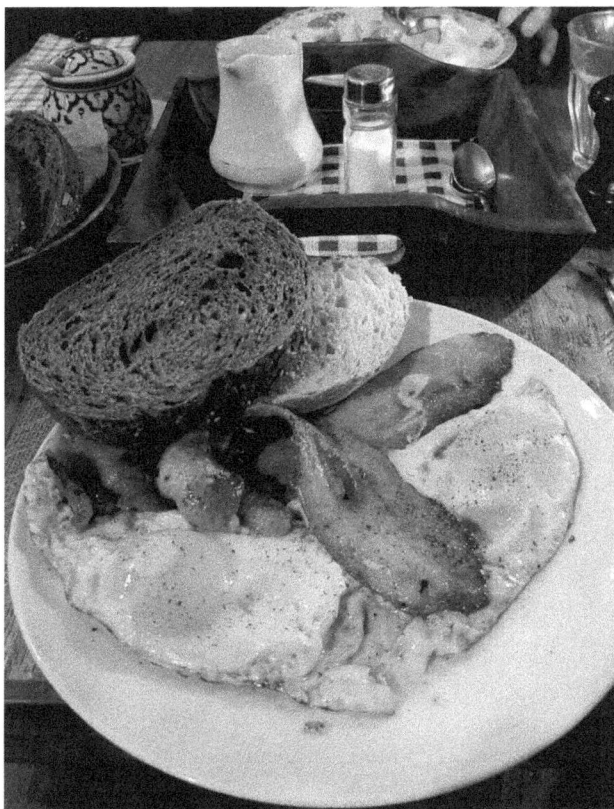

During his investigation, Mosley met up with Walter Willet, a professor at the Harvard School of Public Health, who has been researching about the issues surrounding diet.

"We found that those who consumed higher amounts

of red meat had a higher risk of total mortality, cardiovascular mortality and cancer mortality," Willet told Mosley.

Suzanne Wu, the director of research communications at University of Southern California, had a scary message for Americans one morning in March, 2014.

Wu ran this headline: Meat and cheese may be as bad as smoking.

Reporting on a USC study, Wu wrote in the article that "eating a diet rich in animal proteins during middle age makes you four times more likely to die of cancer than someone with a low-protein diet," adding that this was a factor much like smoking.

Oops.

Soda

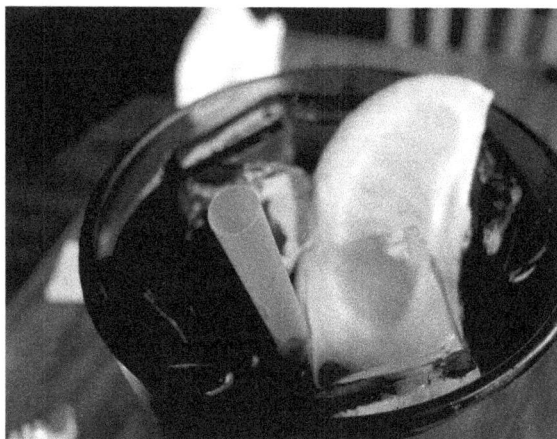

Photo Credit: Nate Brelsford.

Oh, the fresh and cool taste of soda on a hot summer day.

Put that down.

According to Reader's Digest, from their book *Kitchen Cabinet Cures*, there are good reasons to avoid soda, including diet soda. "People who drink sodas instead of healthy beverages (think low-fat milk and pure fruit juice) are less likely to get adequate vitamin A, calcium, and magnesium," says the magazine.

Other reasons?

There is a toxic chemical called bisphenol A (BPA), which can leak from soda (and water) bottles and into your drink and into your body.

If you're like me, and you used to drink diet soda thinking it will help you to lose weight, the magazine says think again. Apparently, diet soda makes you gain weight, too.

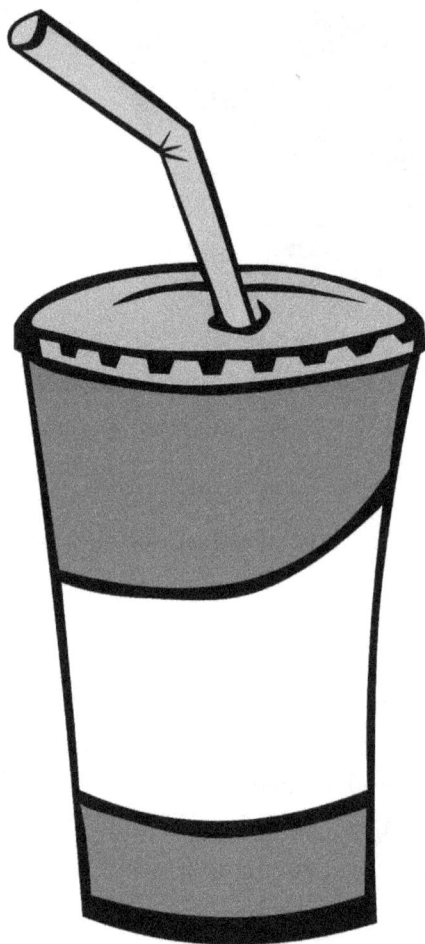

One study showed that people who drank diet soda have about 41% increased risk of gaining weight. It has to do with how our bodies look at anything sweet, as the body stores fat and carbohydrates.

Finally, sodas that contain "high-fructose corn syrup also contain high levels of free radicals linked to tissue damage, the development of diabetes, and diabetic complications," say the magazine.

The magazine put soda on the bad list of their "15 Foods You Should Never Buy Again," too. It also was featured in an article that said, "Diet Soda May Increase the Risk of Stroke."

In other words, stick with healthier drinks.

Breaking The Fast

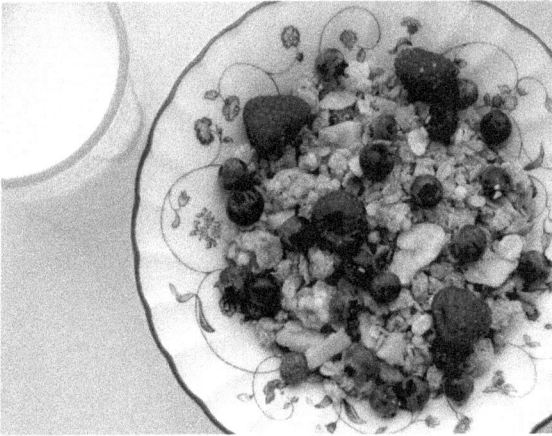

Photo Credit: Marta Rostek.

Think about the word *breakfast*. It is composed of break and fast. In other words, this is a meal that breaks the fast of not having eaten anything since the night before.

Many people skip breakfast. I used to be on one of these people, only having a coffee or water before lunch. Sometimes, generally on Sundays, I did do brunch.

One day, just around 11:30 in the morning, I felt dizzy. I instinctively knew to eat something, and that dizziness slowly dissipated.

"You can't skip breakfast," my doctor warned me, when I visited her a week later to tell her about my experience. "Your body needs to eat every so often, and when you sleep as normally as you should, then your body needs to break that fast in the morning," she added. "Skipping breakfast has many drastic health consequences."

So, I don't skip breakfast anymore.

Benefits of Breakfast

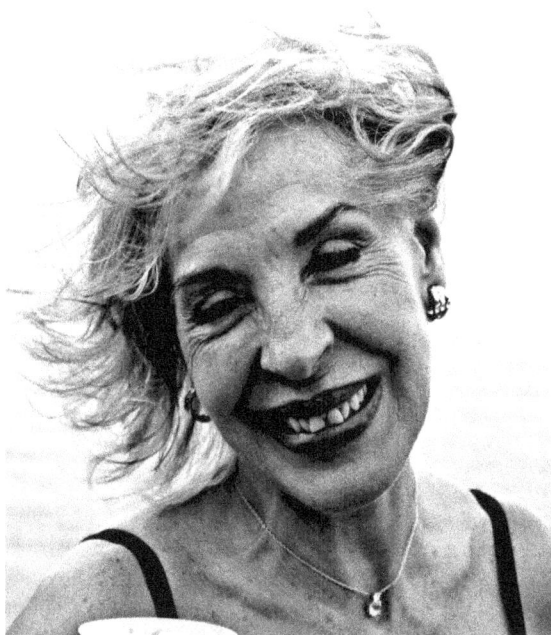

Photo Credit: Hector Landaeta.

When I started eating breakfast, I did feel different. Sometimes, the differences were very little or were connected to things I didn't do everyday.

For example, one time I noticed when I reached for my bike, my stomach felt different. It is hard to explain, but it felt looser.

Of course, after starting eating breakfast again, the first thing I wanted to know was what exactly were the benefits of eating breakfast.

"The most important benefit is energy," said my doctor. "Breakfast gives the body that boost of energy, what it needs to jumpstart its day."

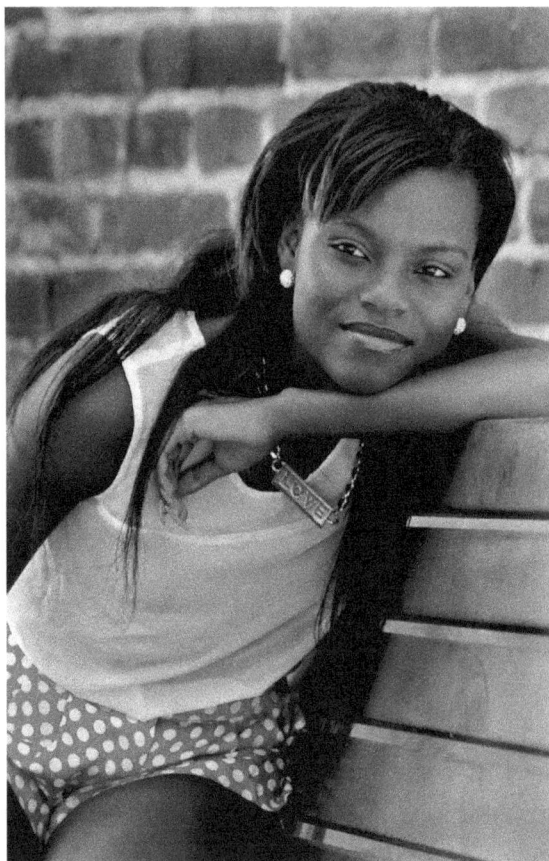

Sheah Rarback, a registered dietitian with the University of Miami's Leonard M. Miller School of Medicine, says enhanced vitamin and mineral intake, weight control, and clearer thinking is some of the benefits of breakfast.

Mike Stobbe, with *USA Today*, wrote about a study by

researchers at Harvard who discovered that breakfast decreased heart attack. The study found 27% higher risk in older men who regularly skipped the meal. The researchers said there was no reason why this wouldn't apply to other age or sex groups.

Best Breakfast

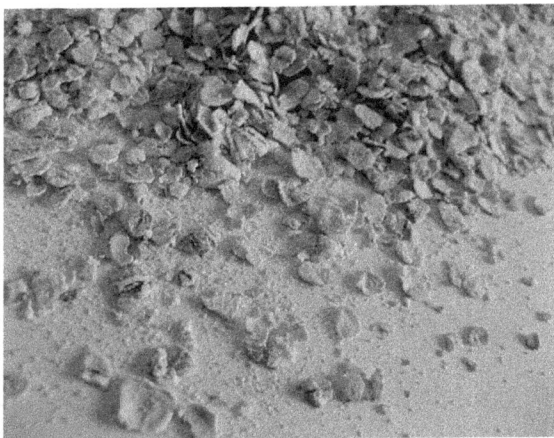

Photo Credit: Valerie Like.

After learning the benefits of breakfast, I, of course, wanted to know what were the best kinds of breakfast.

"Definitely not eggs and bacon every morning," says my doctor. "You want a healthy breakfast, because you want to give your body the chance to work on bettering itself, and giving you good energy, rather than wasting its energy on fixing what you had just fed it."

Erica Giovinazzo, a certified nutritionist at Clay Health Club and Spa in New York City, says that the best breakfast is one that combines good carbs and fiber with some protein.

Oatmeal, Greek yoghurt, and a piece of fruit are what I often eat for breakfast. Generally, I will have a half of banana with my breakfast. Some mornings, I will have one egg. Other mornings, I will have a fresh grapefruit juice with my breakfast.

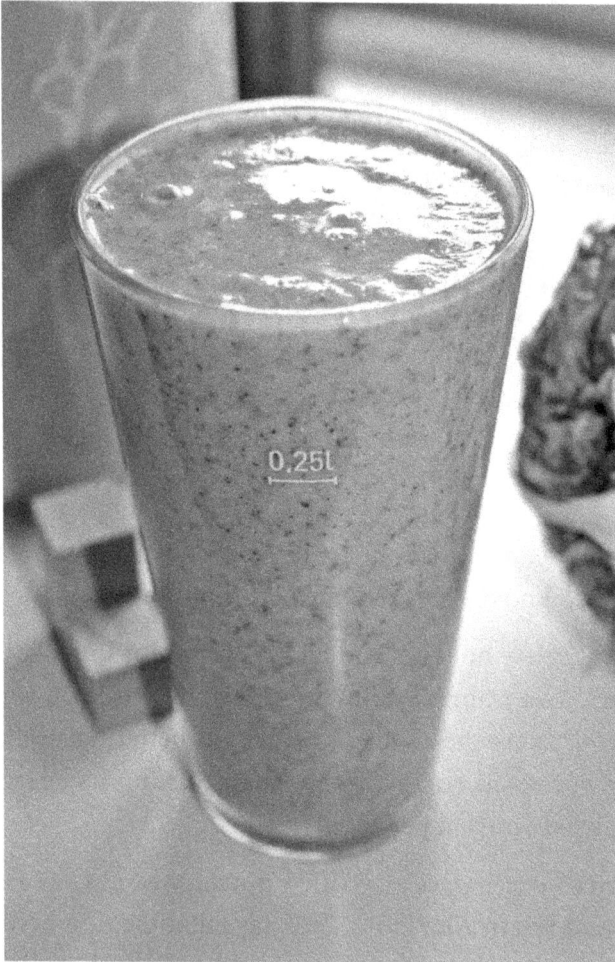

Oatmeal is a great choice. A cup of oatmeal is loaded with 4 grams of fiber, and a half banana brings in another 1 to 1.5 grams.

According to Kathleen M. Zelman, a director of nutrition for *WebMD*, soluble fiber, which is the kind of fiber you would find in both oatmeal and bananas, has many benefits such as lowering the bad cholesterol, regulating blood sugar, and lowering risk of heart disease and type 2 diabetes.

Plus, you can make oatmeal is different ways, including making it into a smoothie (like you see in the photo on the previous page).

Best Time for Breakfast

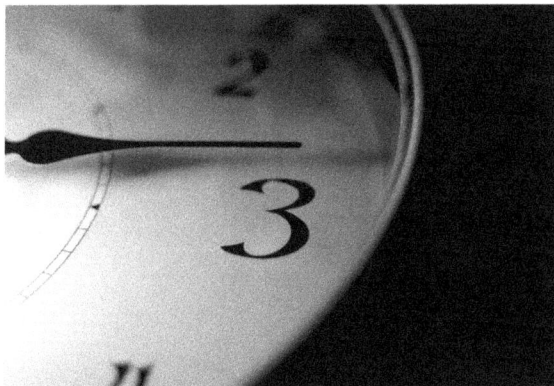

Photo Credit: Chris Gilbert.

Now that you understand the importance of breakfast, the next natural question to ask is exactly when is the best time to eat your breakfast. Well, that all depends on several factors.

According to Michelle Kerns, who covers stories about health for the *San Francisco Chronicle*, a 2011 US Agriculture report, which used 15 studies for its reporting, said that breakfast is a meal taken before 10 in the morning.

That said, it is really about when you wake up.

"Eat within 1 hour of rising," says Natasha Turner, a leading naturopathic doctor and the author of *The Hormone Diet*, and recommends eating every 3 to 4 hours thereafter, stressing on the fact that skipping breakfast would make it "more likely to eat unbalanced meals, more calories, and larger amounts of saturated fat throughout the day."

On the other hand, some have pinpointed the exact time breakfast is most ideal.

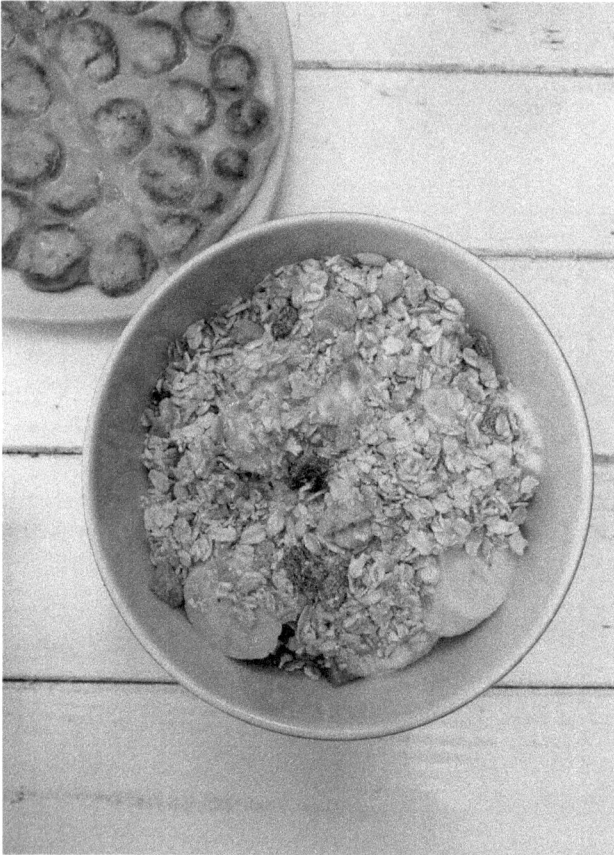

In 2014, a UK-based company that makes dietary supplements called Forza Supplements released a research they conducted from 1000 individuals. "We found that the optimum times were 7.11am for breakfast," Lee Smith, the company's manager director, told the *Daily Mail*.

So, if you are following this program and woke up at 6am, and had your 30-45 minutes of physical activity, then you should be ready to have your breakfast around that time anyway.

Go for it!

Breakfast Recipe

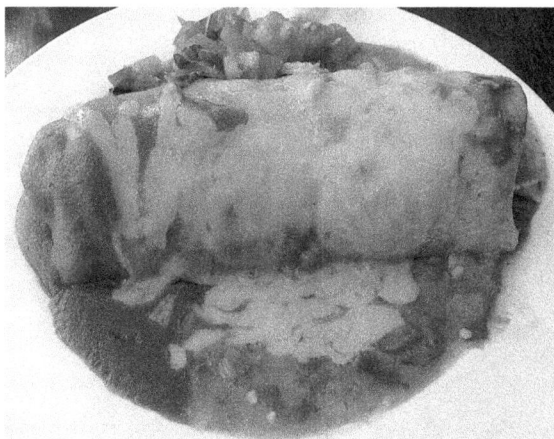

Photo Credit: Alan Levine.

I love recipes. I will be sharing with you recipes throughout the book, about particular meals that I think make this type of lifestyle dieting an easy thing.

So, here's a good recipe that I absolutely love. You never have to twist my arm about burritos. I adore them.

"Breakfast burritos are perfect," said one of my friends, after I made us breakfast using the following recipe.

The following recipe is from the United States Department of Agriculture's *Healthy Eating on a Budget Cookbook*, which is made with funding allocated for the Supplemental Nutrition Assistance Program or SNAP.

It takes 30 minutes to make it, and makes 4 servings. It has 240 calories, 8g fat, 30g of carbohydrate, and 11g of protein.

It is healthy and delicious!

Enjoy!

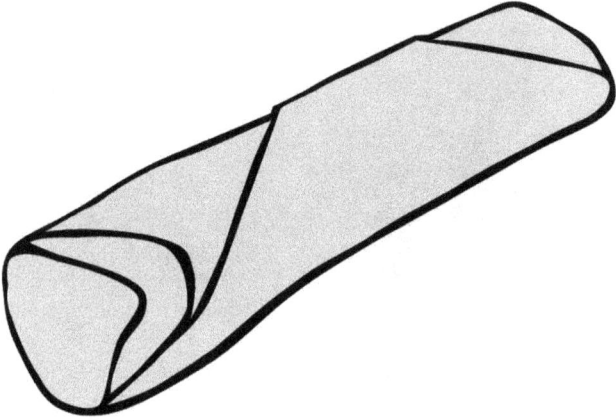

Breakfast Burrito with Salsa

Ingredients

4 eggs (large)

2 tablespoons corn (frozen)

1 tablespoon of milk (1%)

2 tablespoons green pepper (diced)

1/4 cup of onion (minced)

1 tablespoon tomatoes (diced fresh)

1 teaspoon mustard

1/4 teaspoon garlic (granulated)

1/4 teaspoon hot pepper sauce (optional)

4 flour tortillas (8 inch)

1/4 cup salsa (canned)

Directions

Preheat oven to 350 degrees.

1. In a large mixing bowl, blend the eggs, corn, milk, green peppers, onions, tomatoes, mustard, garlic, hot pepper sauce, and salt for 1 minute until eggs are smooth.

2. Pour egg mixture into a lightly oiled 9x9x2 inch baking dish and cover with foil.

3. Bake for 20-25 minutes until eggs are set and thoroughly cooked.

4. Wrap tortillas in plastic and microwave for 20 seconds until warm. Be careful when unwrapping the tortillas. The steam can be hot.

5. Cut baked egg mixture into 4 equal pieces and roll 1 piece of cooked egg in each tortilla.

6. Serve each burrito topped with 2 Tablespoons of salsa.

Snack The Right Way

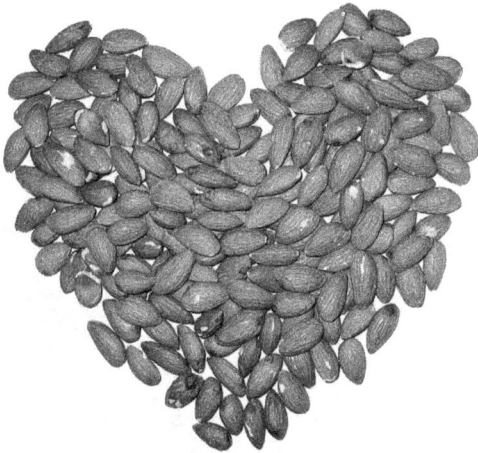

Photo Credit: Maria Li.

So, it was in December of 2011 when a study published in the Journal of the American Dietetic Association shocked the world. The study, which was conducted at the Fred Hutchinson Cancer Research Center in Seattle, said that mid-morning snacking was making it hard to lose weight.

Oops.

Well, this research was totally contradicting the many others before that said snacking was a good thing. Needless to say, it created media frenzy and the blogosphere was on fire.

Fast forward to July of 2013. At the Institute of Food

Technologists (IFT) Annual Meeting & Food Expo in Chicago, researchers from the United Kingdom presented something else. Roberta Re, a researcher and the nutrition research manager at Leatherhead Food Research in Surrey, said snacking was still good if done right.

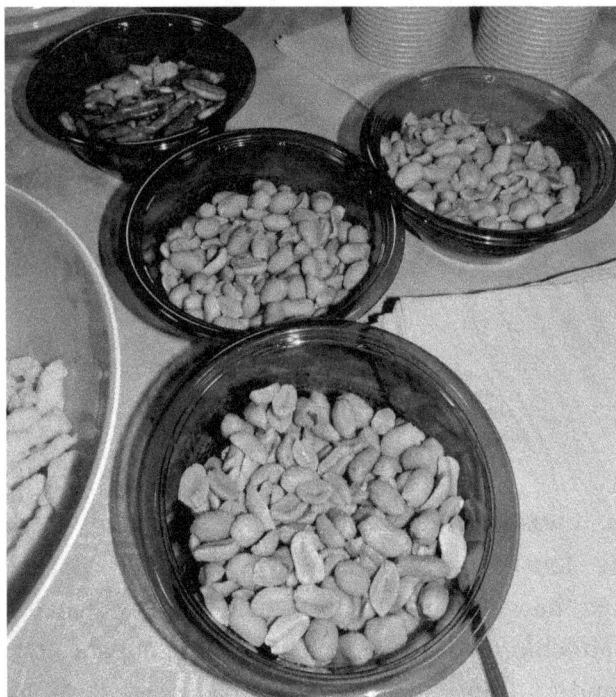

"The main finding of the study on snacking is that consumption of nuts (almonds and peanuts in particular) can help to a reduced subjective perception of appetite and reduce energy intake at the next meal," Re told Marie Benz, a medical doctor who runs the popular *MedicalResearch.com* website, adding that the effect of nuts on satiety has been extensively investigated.

Interestingly enough, just three months before Re and her team presented their research, another research published in the American Journal of Clinical Nutrition basically presented something similar.

"We performed a systematic review and meta-analysis of published, randomized nut-feeding trials to estimate the effect of nut consumption on adiposity measures," wrote researchers from five different universities in Spain, who conducted the study together.

What did they find? That diets enriched with nuts did not increase body weight, body mass index, or waist circumference. In other words, they found the nuts to be healthy.

Best Snacks

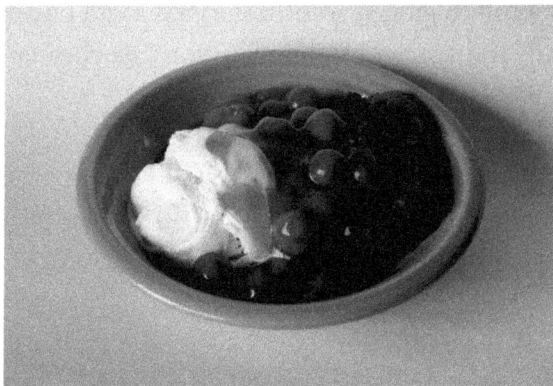

Photo Credit: David Tipton.

Now that you understanding snacking is a good idea if you do it the right way, you're probably wanting to know what types of snacks make it to the best list.

To answer that question, *Health* magazine asked a few experts. Rania Batayneh, author of *The One One One Diet*, Georgie Fear, co-author of *Racing Weight Cookbook: Lean, Light Recipes for Athletes*, and Gayl Canfield, Director of Nutrition at the Pritikin Longevity Center were enlisted.

What did they recommend? Things like Greek yogurt, raspberries, blueberries, bananas, apples, grapes, oranges, walnuts, soynuts, edamame, cottage cheese, cucumbers, olives, and hummus.

Those of you who are craving other types of snacks, don't worry these ladies got your back. They also recommended KIND healthy grains bar, Freekeh foods, Ips' all natural egg white chips, and even Arctic Zero frozen desserts.

How?!? Because of all those things are less than 200 calories. So, indulging is a lot less risky, taste buds are more satisfied, and you end feeling like you just cheated or something!

Best Time to Snack

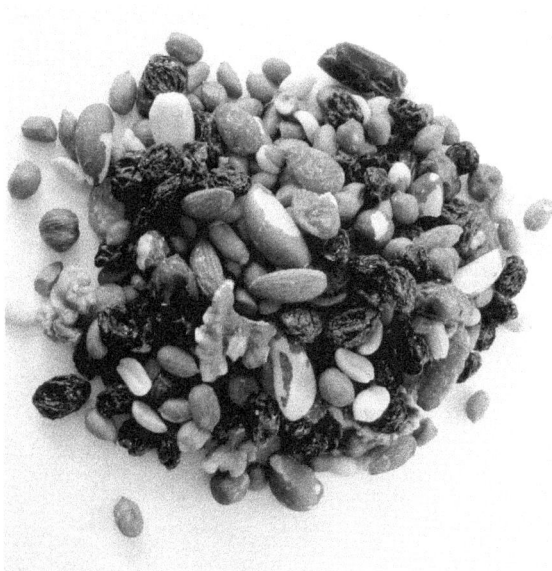

Photo Credit: Chris Chidsey.

If you're going to go for four hours between meals, you need to snack in between says Sarah-Jane Bedwell, a nutritionist for *Self* magazine and the author of *Schedule Me Skinny*.

If you go over four hours without eating, says Bedwell, then your "metabolism will slow down, your blood sugar will drop, and by the time you finally do eat, you will be so ravenous that it will be hard to make good choices and you will be at risk of overeating."

So, basically, that is the general gist. Keep that in mind, and you will be good. Now, are there good times when one should actually snack? It depends, again.

Keri Gans, a nutritionist who helped with *Shape* magazine's 2012 Weight Loss Diary and is the author of *The Small Change Diet*, early risers should snack between breakfast and lunch. In the afternoon, Gans argues, a mid afternoon snack is a must, as it will keep you from overeating later.

Snack Recipe

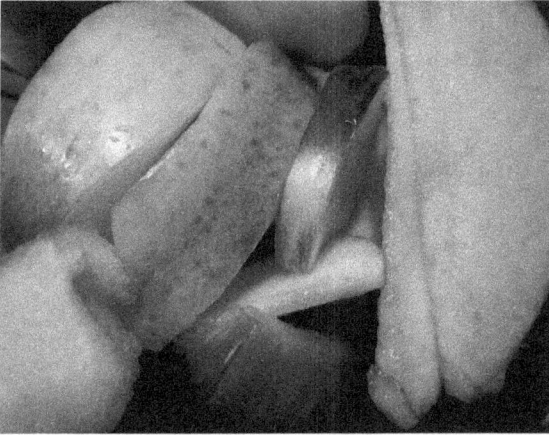

Photo Credit: Andrew Malone.

Apple cinnamon bars are heavenly snacks! They are healthy, and they are not so heavy; yet, they really do satisfy any craving!

Here, once again, we have a recipe from the USDA's *Healthy Eating on a Budget Cookbook*. This recipe makes 24 servings, which each has about 100 calories, 4.5g of fat, 14g of carbohydrate, and 1g of protein.

Apple Cinnamon Bars

Ingredients

4apple (medium)

1 cup of flour

1/4 teaspoon salt

1/2 teaspoon baking soda

1/2 teaspoon cinnamon

1/2 cup brown sugar

1 cup oats (uncooked)

1/2 cup shortening

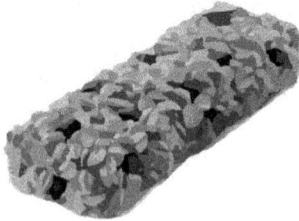

Directions

1. Preheat the oven to 350 degrees.

2. Put the flour, salt, baking soda, cinnamon, brown sugar, and oats in the mixing bowl. Stir together.

3. Add the shortening to the bowl. Use the 2 table knives to mix the ingredients and cut them into crumbs.

4. Lightly grease the bottom and sides of the baking dish with a little bit of shortening.

5. Spread half of the crumb mixture in the greased baking dish.

6. Remove the core from the apples and slice them. Put the apple

slices into the baking dish.

7. Top the apples with the rest of the crumb mixture.

8. Bake in the oven for 40 – 45 minutes.

9. Cut into squares. It will fall apart easily.

The Power Of Lunch

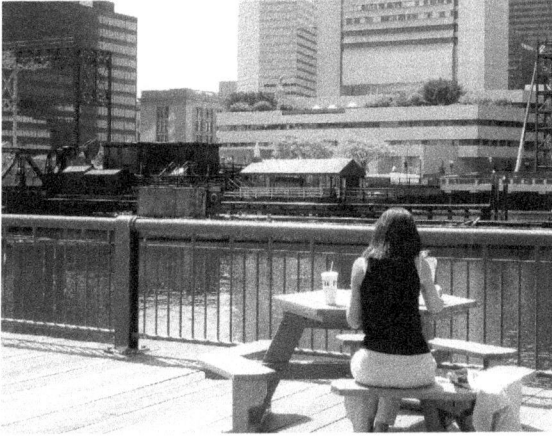

Photo Credit: Muriel Miralles de Sawicki.

I will admit that I love lunch. I have always loved lunch. I might have skipped breakfast, but I never missed my lunch if I could help it.

For most people, even if they eat lunch, don't take actual breaks to go eat it. During September and October of 2012, ManPower's *Right Management*, polled 1,023 North American workers and asked if they regularly took a break for lunch. Guess what, they found that 81% don't take real lunch breaks.

Oops.

Benefits of Lunch

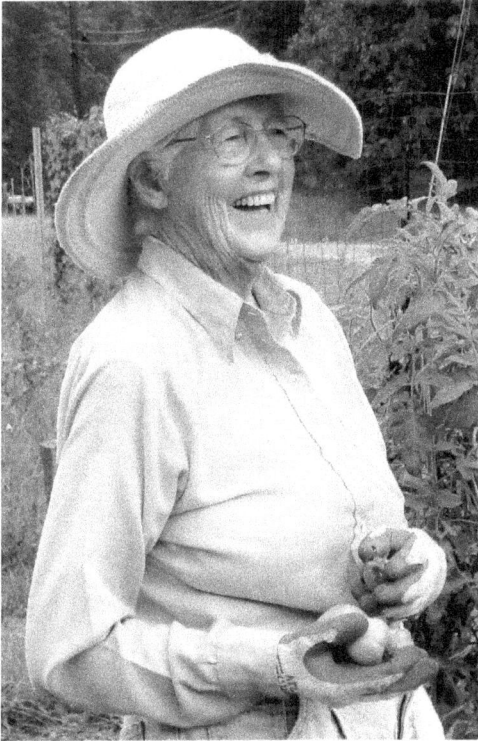

Photo Credit: Carol Garbiano.

Skipping lunch is not a good idea. A benefit of eating lunch, therefore, includes losing weight. "Extended periods of starvation between large meals creates gaps which keep metabolism from staying active," Kurt Hong, M.D., told Huntington Medical Foundation's *HMF Newsletter*. "Your body assumes the worst—there is no more food! It compensates by slowing down," adding that it wouldn't expand energy.

But it is not just eating the lunch, but also being mindful of the lunch. Most of us don't have the chance to pick our own lunch from the garden, but did you know that thinking about where your lunch came from could help you lose weight?

Neither did I!

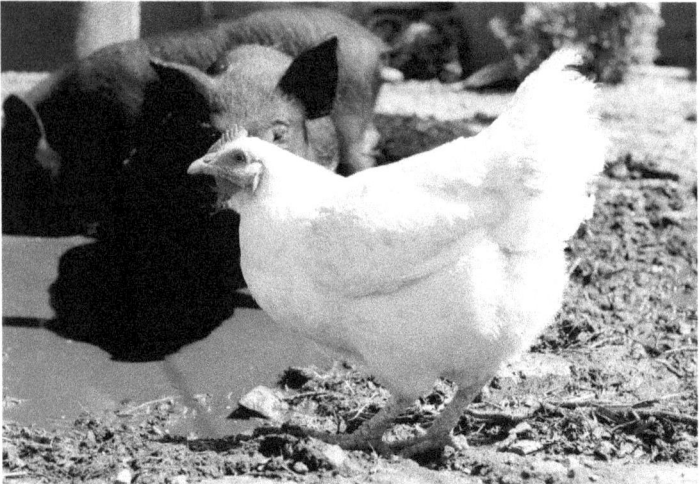

According to Howard LeWine, M.D., the Chief Medical Editor of *Harvard Health Publications*, distracted eating can make you gain weight; and one of the suggested things is to think five minutes about where your food came from, eating silently.

"Paying attention to a meal was linked to eating less later on," wrote LeWine, of studies about eating and weight loss, adding that mindfulness can be practiced throughout daily activities including eating.

How do you do this? LeWine suggests thinking, "what it took to produce that meal, from the sun's rays to the farmer to the grocer to the cook."

LeWine also suggested having a timer on for a 20-minute eating a normal-sized meal, to eat with the non-dominant hand, to take small bites and chew them well, and to ask if one is really hungry before even opening that fridge.

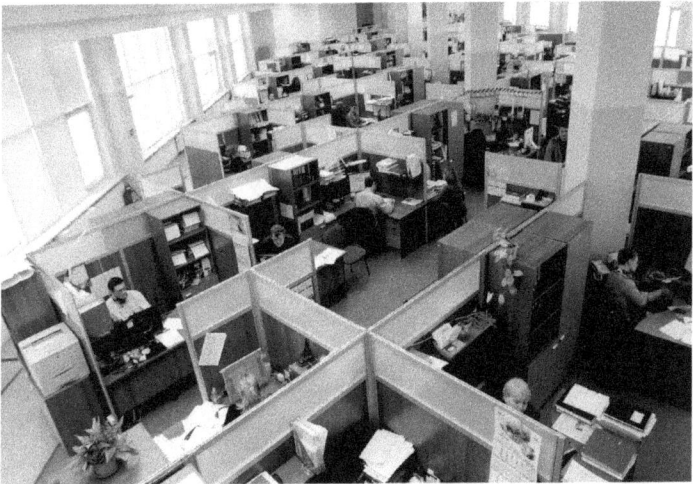

Another benefit of lunch is productivity. Eating your lunch at your desk doesn't count, because it goes against the above advice of avoiding distracted eating. So, taking a lunch break does the business actually better than the other way around.

"Never taking a break from very careful thought work actually reduces your ability to be creative," Kimberly Elsbach, a professor at UC-Davis who studies the psychology of the workplace, told *Time* magazine.

Elsbach explains that not taking a break exhausts your cognitive capacity; leading you to make less creative connections than if your brain was rested.

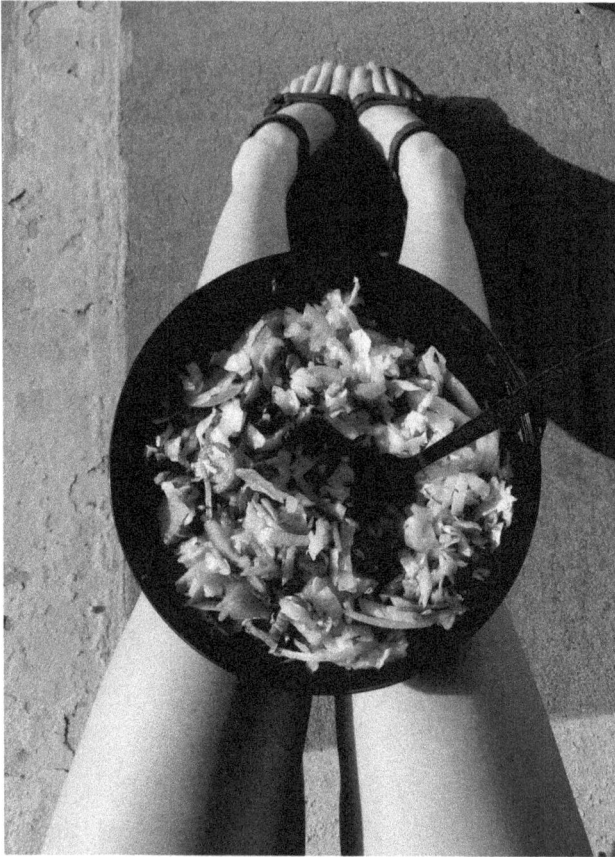

Another benefit of lunch is that it gives us a chance to get a dose of the sun. The phrase "picnic lunch" is an American idea that stands the test of times. It is such a popular idea that on Google the search for the phrase returns about 1,690,000 results (in 0.41 seconds).

A randomized controlled trial by the *British Journal of Dermatology* found that by exposing people to an artificial light, similar to what a person would get from a 10-minute exposure in noon in the summer, that it was sufficient to maintain summer vitamin D levels.

"The UV dose used in this study is equal to two hours and 20 minutes outside under the weak winter sun," wrote Emily Main of *Rodale News*, adding that it "equals 10 minutes of sun exposure a day over the course of two weeks."

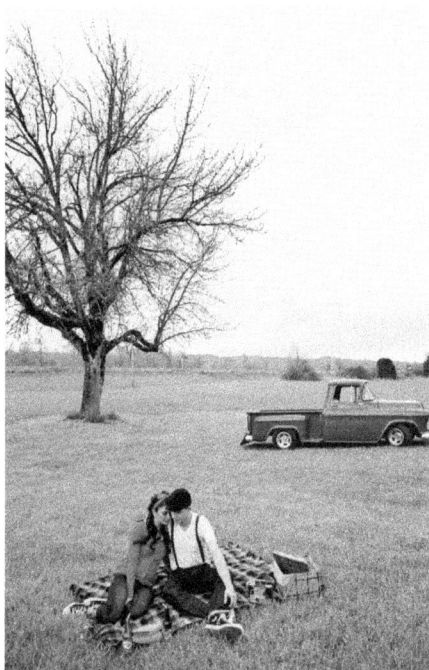

Finally, one more benefit of lunch is that it gives you chances to be social. After having a 20-minute uninterrupted eating, you might have just enough time left from your break to head to Facebook or Twitter to catch up with your friends and family.

According to KISSmetrics, a San Francisco-based company that tracks online activities, people Tweet or share things on Facebook most during lunch hour, as well as in the early evening around.

Of course, you might also decide to meet your significant other or a friend for lunch, and spend all of that time eating and happy!

Best Lunch

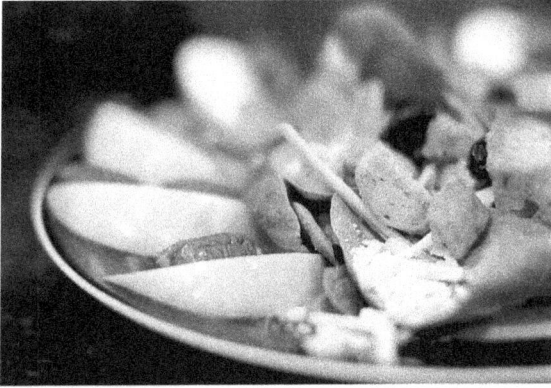

Photo Credit: Jason Miller.

What is the best lunch?

Well, of course, the answer to that depends on whom you ask.

Back in 2008, the European Union had received around 44 thousand health claims from their member states. Tasked with deciding which ones were really healthy, the scientists at the European Food Safety Authority (EFSA) had spent five years to bring that down to just 222.

Leatherhead Food Research, a marketing and research company for the food industry located just outside of London, had come up with a meal that incorporates all of those 222 health claims approved by the European Union.

What does such a meal look like? The meal, named the *Leatherhead Airline Meal Formula 222*, includes smoked salmon terrine, mixed leaf salad with olive oil, multi-grain bread, chicken casserole with lentils as well as vegetables, yoghurt blancmange, and sport drink composed of cranberry, raspberry and elderflower.

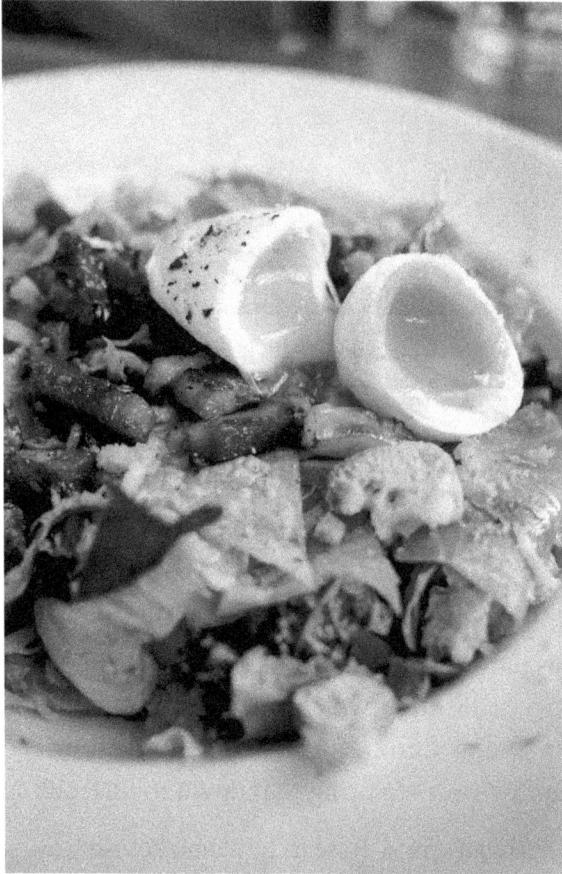

Elaine Magee, a registered nutritionist and the author of *Food Synergy*, says that making "one simple change to your diet – adding a salad almost every day – can pay off with plenty of health benefits," adding that salads have many health benefits such as lowering bad cholesterol, giving us higher blood levels of powerful antioxidants, and simply giving us a chance to eat more good fats such as those found in olive oil.

If you snacked at midmorning, then a good size salad will be the perfect lunch.

Now that we decided on salad as the good option for lunch, what would be a good salad? Joy Bauer, the nutritionist and health expert for NBC's the *Today* show, has set up a 5-point system to help you get the best out of your salad.

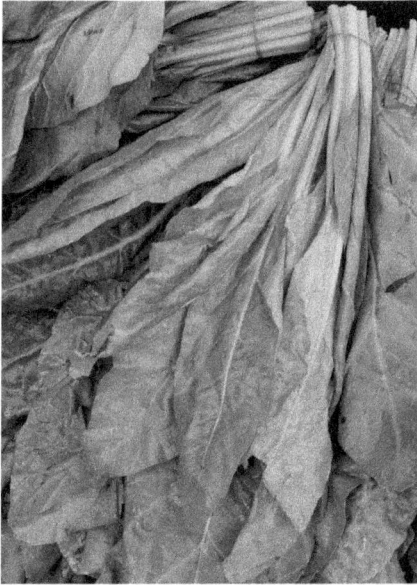

Bauer starts with a recommendation to give up "the iceberg for mesclun greens, baby spinach, or a spring mix that includes a variety of dark green lettuces."

Now that your green base has been chosen, she recommends adding veggies like bell peppers, carrots, broccoli, cucumbers, red onions, or even sugar snap peas.

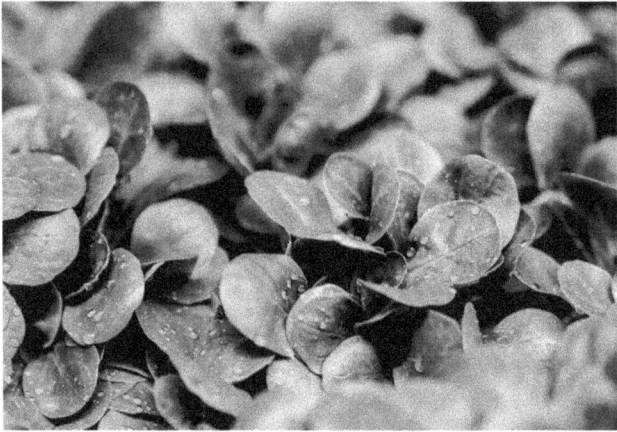

Next, Bauer notes that by adding protein your salad becomes a meal. For non-animal proteins, she recommends tofu, chickpeas, or beans. For animal products, she says to choose one lean source or two if you're really hungry.

After having your greens, vegetables, and proteins all in place, Bauer recommends to sparingly add what she calls extras. "Extras are those items that typically add another dimension and flavor to your combo," she explains.

These extras would include either 2 tablespoons of cheese (cheddar, Parmesan, goat, Swiss, or feta), 1 tablespoon of nuts (walnuts, pecans or almonds), 1 ounce of avocado, 10 small olives (either canned or jarred in water), 1/4 cup of croutons, or 2 tablespoons of dried cranberries or raisins.

Finally, you want to dress up your salad in a healthy way. "One tablespoon of your average vinaigrette is about 80 calories and one tablespoon of creamy ranch is almost 100 calories," she says. Instead, she recommends using her recipe of light balsamic vinaigrette, which only has 59 calories.

To use Bauer's dressing, mix 1/2 cup of good quality balsamic vinegar, 3 tablespoons extra-virgin olive oil, 1/4 cup water, 1 tablespoon Dijon mustard, 1 teaspoon honey, and 1 teaspoon garlic powder in a jar, close it, and shake it really good.

The serving size is 2 tablespoons.

Best Time to Eat Lunch

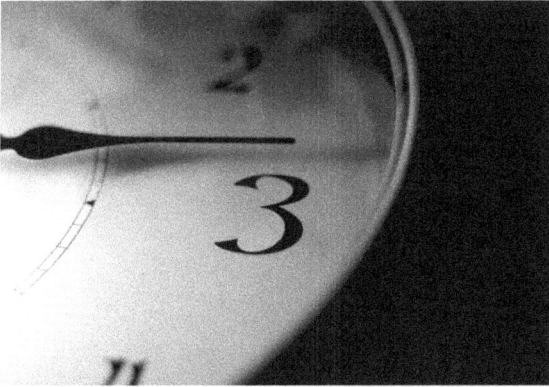

Photo Credit: Chris Gilbert.

Back at breakfast we came to the calculation that for this program you would have your breakfast around 7am.

Then Natasha Turner, a leading naturopathic doctor and the author of *The Hormone Diet*, recommended eating every 3 to 4 hours thereafter, which means you had your snack around 9:30 to 10am, which pin points your lunch to around noon to 12:30pm.

In December of 2010, Dr. Oz teamed up with Sharecare and the Nike SPARQ Training Network to offer 11-week free program he called *Move It to Lose It*. During week five, the participants were met with a 3-part video and a message that said, "Are you having trouble losing weight? It is not what you're doing; it is when you're doing it. Learn the best time to fight fat."

In the part 2 video, Dr. Oz is talking to a woman who

woke up early but didn't have her breakfast until 9am, ate her lunch at 1pm, and who had her dinner usually around 6pm.

"If you wake up at 6:30," said Dr. Oz, "you should have breakfast at around 7:30, within an hour of" waking up, adding that lunch should be had at noon.

By having your lunch at the right time, you will be able to sustain the energy your body had gained from breakfast and from your midmorning snack.

Lunch Recipe

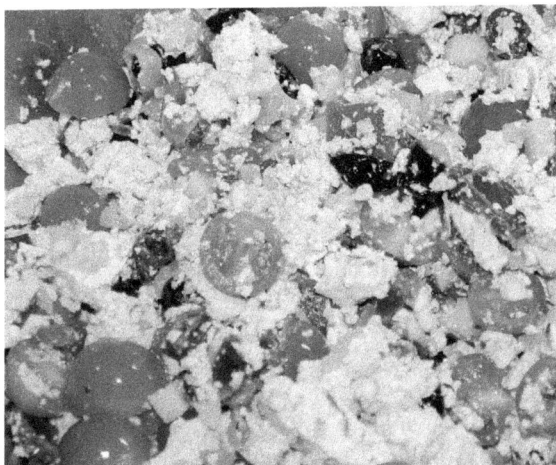

Photo Credit: Scott Veg.

You already got Joy Bauer's amazing salad recipe, but if you want to try something else (and you didn't have eggs for breakfast), perhaps you will love this great scrambled tofu.

Once again, we have a recipe from the USDA's *Healthy Eating on a Budget Cookbook*. This recipe makes 4 servings, and each has about 140 calories, 10g of fat, 1g of carbohydrate, and 13g of protein.

If you add, like I always do, 1 slice of whole wheat bread, it will end up adding 69 calories, 1g of fat, 12g of carbohydrate, and 4g of protein to your over all intake.

Scrambled Tofu

Ingredients

1 package tofu (20 ounces)

1 tablespoon butter

2 eggs

Salt and pepper (optional, to taste)

Bean sprouts or chop suey mix, garlic, watercress, mushrooms, cheese, bell pepper, green onions (optional)

Directions

1. Drain tofu.

2. In small bowl, dice or mash tofu. For optional ingredients, crush garlic and/or slice watercress, mushrooms, cheese, bell peppers, and green onions.

3. In a pan, melt butter. Add tofu. Add optional ingredients. Saute over medium heat until lightly browned.

4. Beat eggs and add to tofu mixture. Cook until firm.

5. Sprinkle with salt and pepper to taste.

6. Stir and cook until firm.

Siesta In the Afternoon

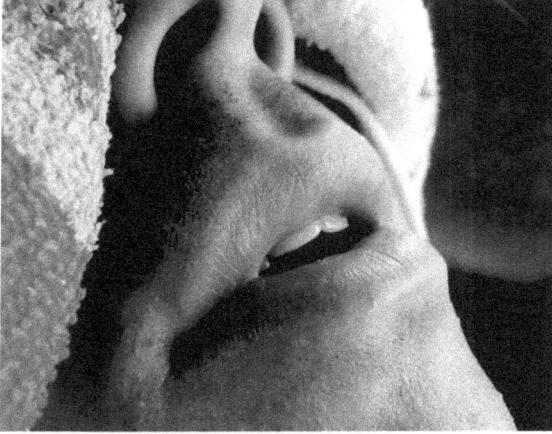

Photo Credit: Maja Lampe.

"Siesta" is a Spanish word that basically translates as "nap."

Do you nap?

Well, I certainly did not. But, did you know that around 85% of mammals nap regularly? According to the Sleep Foundation, most mammals are "polyphasic sleepers, meaning that they sleep for short periods throughout the day. Humans are part of the minority of monophasic sleepers, meaning that our days are divided into two distinct periods, one for sleep and one for wakefulness."

Okay, so they don't exactly nap once. I should have said that they don't sleep all at once. I don't think I could do it, to tell you the truth. I would be crazy all day.

Napping, if you will, is then a compromise. It says we sleep most of the night, but we take a short break that gives us a boost in the middle of the daylight hours.

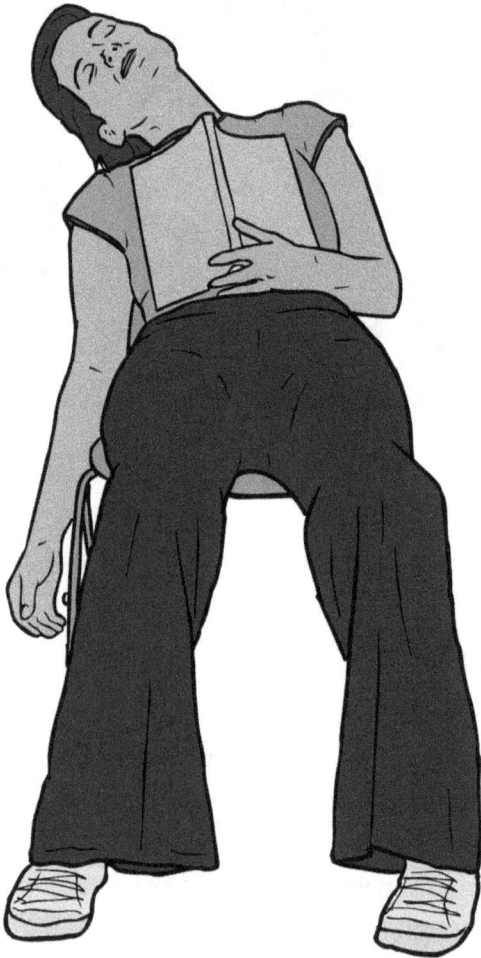

In the United States, thanks to Cornell University social psychologist James Maas, we are familiar with the power nap, a short 10-15 minute sleep. This came about when we realized we are a nation that is sleep deprived. Recently, in 2013, a Gallup Poll showed that 40% of Americans still get less than 7 hours of sleep.

In his biography of Charlemagne, *Vita Karoli Magni* (Life of Charles the Great), the Frankish scholar Einhard wrote that Charlemagne would sleep in the afternoon for 2 to 3 hours.

So, napping, it seems, can be from 10 minutes to 3 hours!

Let's go find out why I nap these days.

Benefits of Napping

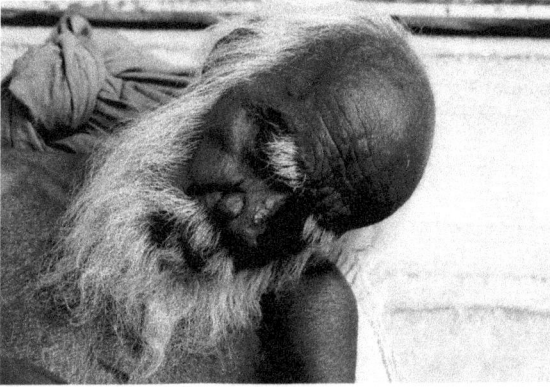

Photo Credit: Manu Mohan.

What if you knew during your afternoons, when your mind and body slow down, that nap could improve your alertness and performance?

That is exactly why I took up napping!

According to the Sleep Foundation, a NASA study found that napping just 40 minutes improved alertness by 100%! Similarly, performance was improved by 34%.

However, benefits of napping go beyond just alertness and performance. According to Sara Mednick, the co-author of *Take a Nap! Change Your Life*, napping is a "necessary and effective tool that can be used by anyone in pursuit of optimum health, happiness and productivity."

We have already learned how napping can help us be more productive, but how can napping be aiding our health and happiness?

Dimitrios Trichopoulos, from the Harvard School of Public Health, led a study on napping published in February of 2007 in the *Archives of Internal Medicine*.

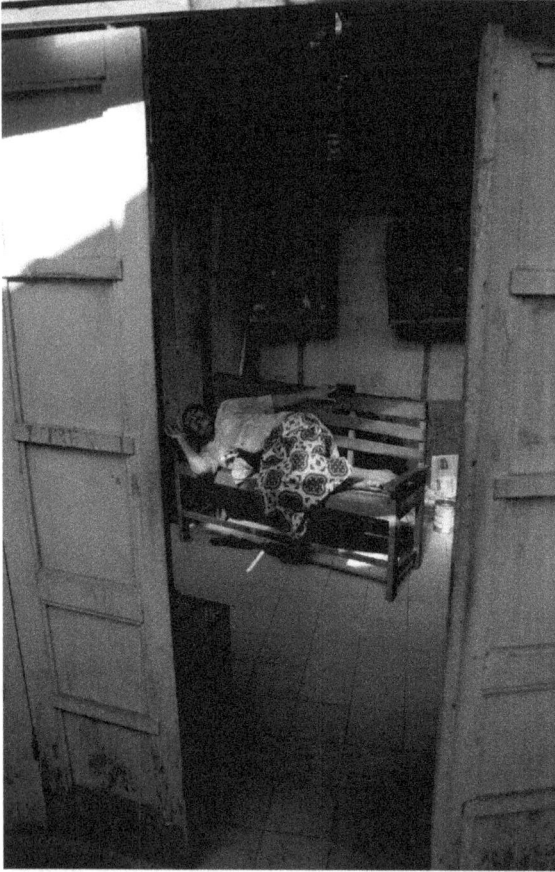

In it, the study revealed how more than 23,000 Greeks were followed, and found that those who did their afternoon siestas were 30% less likely to die of heart disease.

What about happiness?

According to Po Bronson and Ashley Merryman, authors of *NurtureShock: New Thinking About Children*, happiness is all about what you remember. Amygdala is part of the brain that processes negative stimuli, while neutral or positive memories get processed by the hippocampus.

"Sleep deprivation hits the hippocampus harder than the amygdala," wrote Bronson and Merryman on page 35 of their book. "The result is that sleep-deprived people fail to recall pleasant memories, yet recall gloomy memories just fine."

Oops.

Best Nap

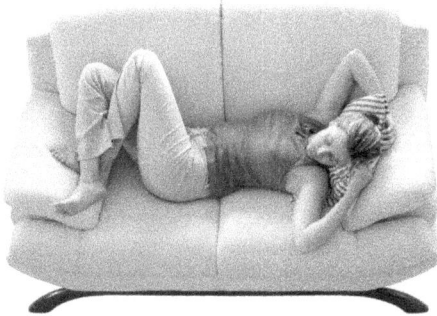

Photo Credit: Piotr Lewandowski.

There are many kinds of naps. Of course, it all depends on you, your day, and, more importantly, what you want to achieve.

According to the Sleep Foundation, napping can be divided into three categories: planned, emergency, and habitual.

Planned napping is a nap you schedule in times you know you won't be sleeping your normal bedtime. That is, if you're going out that night with friends and know you won't be back to your home until 3am this would be the nap you would squeeze in earlier in the day.

Emergency napping is a nap you take when you absolutely cannot go on with your day. If you have worked all night and are on your way home, and you notice you cannot keep your eyes open this would the kind of nap you would be taking right off the highway.

Habitual napping is taking a nap, more or less, around the same time of the day. This is what, for example, the Spanish do with their siestas when their working hours come to a halt in the afternoon for 2 to 3 hours.

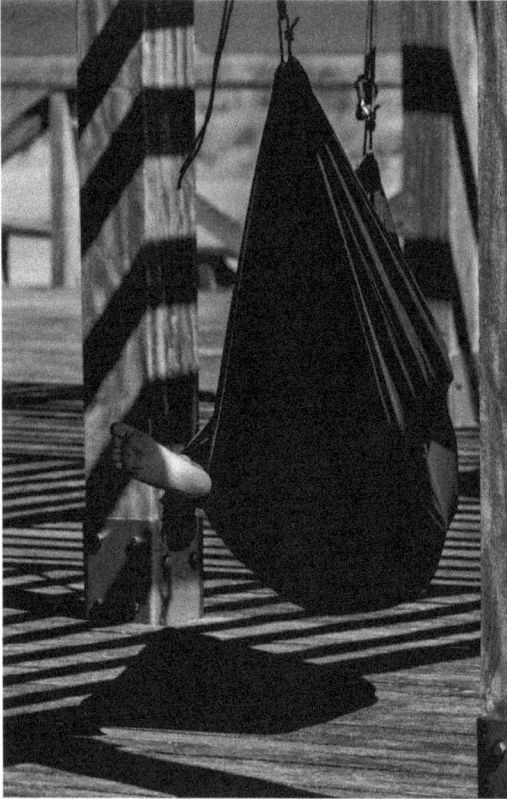

"Napping can steal the drive for nighttime sleep, so you need to be cautious," David Neubauer, M.D., associate director of the Johns Hopkins Sleep Disorders Center, told *Men's Health.* "The key is to nap early and short."

What is early napping? Sara Mednick, who I cited earlier, created Nap Wheel, which is an interactive wheel to help you know exactly when to nap. She says that when you nap totally depends on when you wake up.

"To design your own custom nap, drag the 'wake-up time' dial to the hour you woke up, " she wrote on her website's section for the Nap Wheel. "Follow the hours clockwise until you reach the point in the day when REM and slow-wave sleep cross," she added.

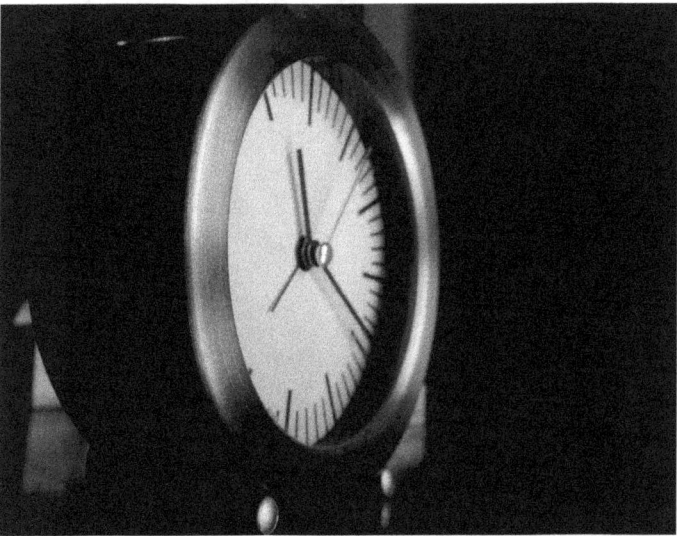

I followed those directions and noticed that if you woke up at 6am then you would have your nap more or less at 1:30pm.

Mednick says the Nap Wheel helps you to find the perfectly balanced state she calls The Ultimate Nap, and that napping before will have more REM and napping after will have more SWS.

But how much time should you nap?

Michael Breus, the author of *Good Night: The Sleep Doctor's 4-Week Program to Better Sleep and Better Health*, says it depends.

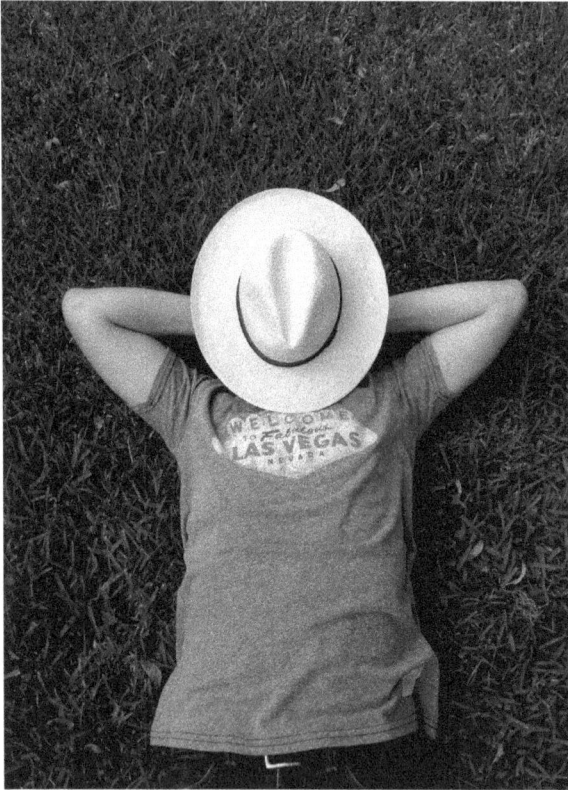

"The [30-minute] nap is particularly important for people who are tired during the day and didn't sleep enough that night, and want to supplement their sleep a little bit," Breus told the *Huffington Post*. "If you take it longer than

30 minutes, you end up in deep sleep."

But deep sleep is not a bad idea, according to Mednick. In 2010, she presented a study at the American Psychological Association's annual convention. She pointed out that people who had 90-minute naps performed better on creativity-oriented word problems.

So, in other words, if you want quick refreshment for your busy day, then the 30-minute nap is best for you. If you were after getting your creative juices rejuvenated, then you would opt for the 90-minute one.

Meditate It All Away

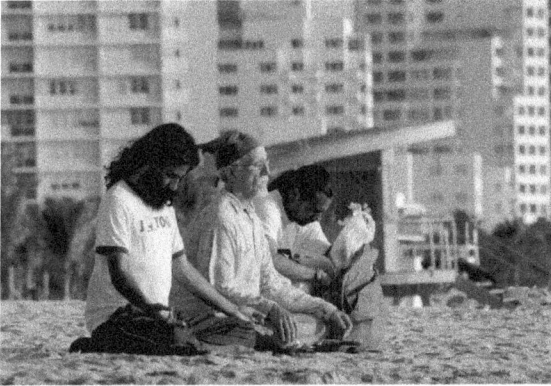

Photo Credit: Ulrik De Wachter.

Stress. Just the word alone makes you feel uneasy. The American Psychological Association's *The Impact of Stress* reports that 7 out of 10 Americans are stressed.

Science has proven that meditation is a good way to combat stress.

In the United States, meditation is a new phenomenon. That is because while napping is a western idea, which we know from Mediterranean cultures, meditation is totally an eastern idea, which is rooted in Hinduism and later in Buddhism, as well as other eastern traditions.

However, like yoga, mediation is becoming more and more accessible to more people. There are many local spiritual centers at which one can learn how to meditate.

I meditate everyday now. I usually meditate in the

morning, and sometimes in the afternoon if I don't have enough time to take a nap, and I can tell you first hand that it changes your life for the better.

Let's look at this amazing adventure.

Benefits of Meditation

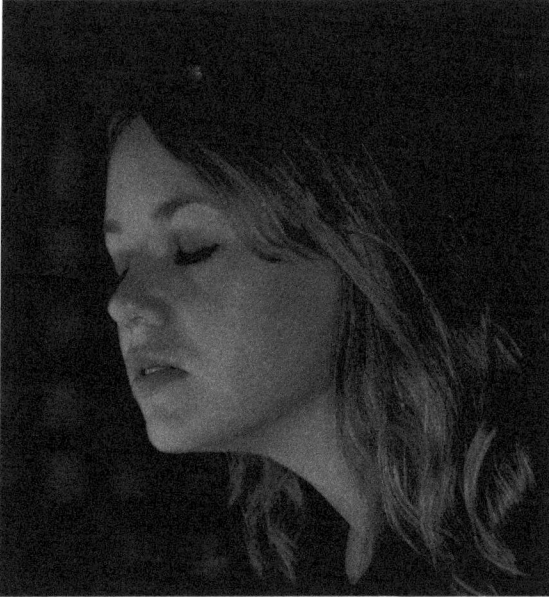

Photo Credit: Anita Peppers.

There are many benefits to meditating, and they all add up to something important: that meditation really promotes happiness.

In 2011, ABC's *Nightline* reported on meditation. "Several studies suggest that these changes through meditation can make you happier, less stressed -- even nicer to other people," wrote ABC's Dan Harris and Erin Brady, adding that it "can help you control your eating habits and even reduce chronic pain, all the while without taking prescription medication."

Harris and Brady basically summed up all that is important about meditation. Everything else in this section will just reiterate that.

In January 2014, Julie Corliss, Executive Editor of the *Harvard Heart Letter*, wrote in her publication that researchers from Johns Hopkins University went through 19,000 meditation studies and that their findings, which published in the Journal of the American Medical Association's *Internal Medicine* in the same month, suggest "that mindfulness meditation can help ease psychological stresses like anxiety, depression, and pain."

Well, 2014 was a big year for meditation and stress studies. In February, the Institute for Natural Medicine and Prevention at Maharishi University in Iowa released a study about how teachers and staff working at a school for children with behavior problems felt their stress were lessened after doing transcendental meditation for 20 minutes.

In May, a study published in the *American Journal of Psychiatry* found that a 20-hour meditational course aimed at military personnel helped those who engaged in the meditation fared better than those who didn't. The researchers said that the results show "mechanisms related to stress recovery can be modified in healthy individuals prior to stress exposure," meaning military personnel could partake in meditation prior to going to stressful war situations.

In July, a study at the Carnegie Mellon University in Pennsylvania, which was published in *Psychoneuroendocrinology*, reported that 25-minute mindfulness meditation alters psychological and neuroendocrine responses to social evaluative stress.

But what about if you're not stressed? Well, for one it can help you prevent colds. One study by University of Wisconsin-Madison followed a group people before and after the winter and found that the adults who practiced meditation had fewer seasonal ailments during the following winter than the ones who did not.

How is that possible? Probably because meditation makes your brain stronger. A study at UCLA in 2012 looked at the MRI scans of meditators and non-meditators, taking existing MRI scans for the control group while the meditators were recruited from meditation venues.

"The meditators had practiced their craft on average for 20 years using a variety of meditation types — Samatha, Vipassana, Zen and more," reported Mark Wheeler in *UCLA Newsroom*, adding that the researchers "found pronounced group differences (heightened levels of gyrification in active meditation practitioners) across a wide swatch of the cortex, including the left precentral gyrus, the left and right anterior dorsal insula, the right fusiform gyrus and the right cuneus."

Interestingly enough, the researchers were able to find a correlation between the number of years an individual meditated and the amount of insular gyrification.

Finally, one big benefit of meditating is that you become a more compassionate person. Researchers from Northeastern University and Harvard University examined the effects meditation would have on compassion and virtuous behavior.

The study invited participants to an 8-week trainings in two types of meditations. After the sessions, they were put to the test:

"Sitting in a staged waiting room with three chairs were two actors. With one empty chair left, the participant sat down and waited to be called," wrote Lori Lennon, Communications Coordinator for Northeastern University, adding that another actor would enter the room, using crutches and pretending to be in physical pain.

As the new actor entered, the other actors in the room would pretend to be ignoring her by playing with their phones.

The study wanted to know if meditators were willing to help.

They did. While only 15% of non-meditators came to the aide of the actress with crutches, 50% meditators helped––showing that meditation indeed helps people become nicer.

Best Meditation

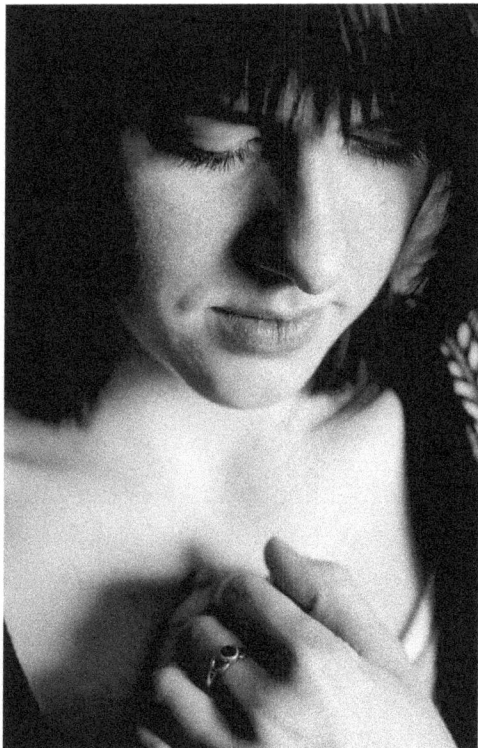

Photo Credit: Jesse Therrien.

Meditation is a practice between science, faith, and culture, depending on how you come across it. As such, it is a very difficult thing to tell someone what is "best."

"As a meditation teacher, I'm frequently asked which type of meditation is the best or the most effective," says Tamara Lechner, a Canadian happiness expert and Primordial Sound Meditation Instructor who has been certified by the Chopra Center, adding "whatever works for you is the right approach, and you have plenty of varieties to choose from."

Lechner describes five styles of meditations as follows: *Primordial Sound Meditation*, which is a type where specifically designed mantra is used; *Mindfulness-Based Stress Reduction*, also known as MBSR, a type that is often administered by health professionals; *Zen*, a traditional Buddhist meditation in which philosophy, practice, and teacher interaction are all part of the equation; *Transcendental Meditation*, also known as TM, in which mantras are used as a way to focus on the meditation; and *Kundalini Yoga*, a type that has hundreds of types that generally require a teacher to specify a tailored kind.

"Different meditation techniques can actually be divided into two main groups," explains Nancy Bazilchuk, a science writer who reported on the subject for the *ScienceDaily*. "One type is concentrative meditation, where the meditating person focuses attention on his or her breathing or on specific thoughts, and in doing so, suppresses other thoughts."

The other, says Bazilchuk, is a kind that is nondirective where the mind is allowed to wander as it pleases, even if the practitioner might say mantras or even listen to audio material.

So, scientifically speaking, which one is better? Researchers at the University of Oslo and the University of Sydney tested a group of meditators and instructed them to rest, meditate concentratively and meditate nondirectively.

The study concluded that nondirective meditation had

higher activity in a part of the brain that deals with personal memories and thoughts.

Svend Davanger, a neuroscientist at the University of Oslo and co-author of the study, told *ScienceDaily* that the "study indicates that nondirective meditation allows for more room to process memories and emotions than during concentrated meditation."

So, it all depends on what you're after. If you want to allow your brain more room to process memories and emotions, then you would want to do a nondirective meditation.

Hold Yourself Over

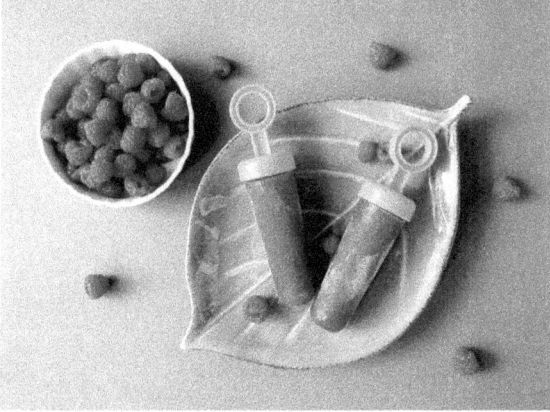

Photo Credit: Jennifer Chait.

You have already read the amazing benefits of snacking. So, whether you napped or meditated, or both, I always recommend an afternoon snack. Afternoon snacks help us to stay energetic until dinnertime.

On hot summer afternoons, nothing is better than a healthy Popsicle! I love, love, love this great recipe. I would suggest popping them in the freezer before you start your day in the morning. That way, when you need them, they are right there!

To keep it healthy, only use 100% juice and good quality yogurt. I personally like to get fresh fruits and make the juicing myself. However, you can find good quality and 100% juices in all major supermarkets these days.

Once again, we have a recipe from the USDA's *Healthy*

Eating on a Budget Cookbook. This recipe makes 4 servings, and each has about 45 calories, 0g of fat, 10g of carbohydrate, and 1g of protein.

Yogurt Pops

Ingredients

6 ounces yogurt, fat-free, flavored or plain

3/4 cup fruit juice

Directions

1. Put the yogurt and juice in a bowl.

2. Stir together well.

3. Pour the mix into paper cups.

4. Stick a Popsicle stick in the center of the mix in the cup.

5. Place the yogurt pops in the freezer until they turn solid.

Dining Before Fast

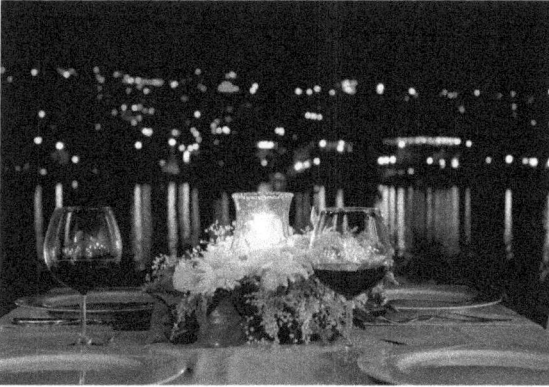

Photo Credit: Emre Nacigil.

Personally I never had any problems with eating dinner. It was and it still is my favorite meal of the day. I admit my dinner habits are a lot healthier these days, but you never to have to twist my arm to enjoy a dinner!

Whether enjoyed with family, friends, a special person, or even with oneself, dinner is definitely an important meal.

Remember Natasha Turner, the naturopathic doctor, and the author of *The Hormone Diet*, who in our breakfast section recommended eating every 3 to 4 hours throughout your day?

Well, dinner is a must because you won't be eating for at least another 7 to 8 hours.

Now that we know it is important, let's tackle the issue and find out why you need to ditch the fast food, frozen dinners, and take-outs for this one.

Benefits of Dinner

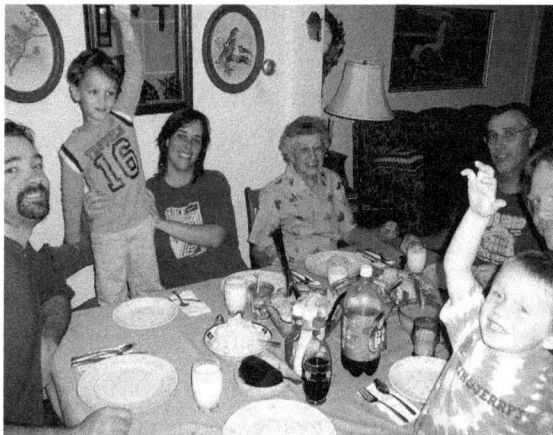

Photo Credit: Mrsmaxspix on Flickr.

Remember family dinners? Being around the table, eating, sharing, talking and just being with family? Remember how sweet it was, to sit on your dad's lap and wave to the camera?

Sadly, more and more families are opting out of family dinners.

"These days, fewer than one-third of all children sit down to eat dinner with both parents on any given night," wrote Cameron Stracher, an NYU Law professor, for *The Wall Street Journal* way back in 2005.

His own personal story was heartbreaking. He was commuting to Manhattan and was not able to get back home before 7:30 or 8, which was too late for his young kids. His wife would sometimes wait for him, and other times he would just eat on the way home in the train.

"60 Years Ago, the average dinnertime was 90 minutes. Today it is less than 12 minutes," writes the Maryland-based *Scramble* website, which helps families plan healthy meals, adding that in "the past 20 years, the frequency of family dinners has declined 33 percent."

Family dinners are one of the benefits of dinner, because it deals with benefits outside of just eating.

"Eating family dinners at least five times a week drastically lowers a teen's chance of smoking, drinking, and using drugs," reported Sarah Klein for the CNN's *Living*, and said that family dinners are cheaper as the costs are "$8 per meal outside of the home, and only about $4.50 per each meal made in your own kitchen."

So, kids on track and saving money are good benefits to dinner. Apparently, dinners also can be a good way to keep your relationship on track.

Cory Allen, a licensed Marriage and Family Therapist and the co-host of *Sexy Marriage Radio*, writes on his website, *Simple Marriage*, that "if you make a point of eating together, you will automatically be creating the shared time so critical for ensuring you don't drift apart."

Aside from connecting, other benefits noted by Allen include the fact that dinners together provide a chance to be grateful, eat mindfully, relax, and even have fun.

People who eat together "tend to eat more vegetables and fruits -- and fewer fried foods, soda, and foods with trans fats, research shows," writes Jeanie Lerche Davis, the winner of a World Wide Web Award for health, for *WebMD*, and recommends avoiding television or answering phones during dinner.

Best Dinner

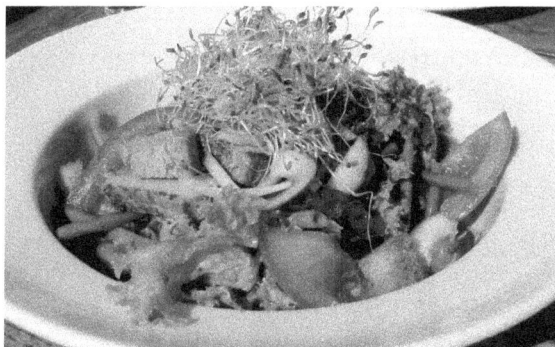

Photo Credit: Knut Pettersen.

Now that we know the benefits of dinner, what kind of dinners should we be eating?

Susan White, a nutritionist who wrote for the UK-based *Mental Healthy*, says that the right dinner can get the body power.

"Ensuring that there is a steady supply of glucose for the body to use as fuel for essential processes whilst we sleep is critical," says White.

For that, White suggests to combine protein and carbohydrates in your dinner. She says if you end up lacking glucose you might end up waking up in the middle of the night, and might not be able to easily go back to sleep.

Dinner can give us better mood and well-being. By eating the right food, White says, dinner can help us to get the right neurotransmitters to work on our behalf.

Serotonin, for example, is derived from the conversion of certain foods that contain tryptophan, an amino acid, such as chicken, turkey, tuna, as well as nuts, seeds, and bananas.

"It is worth remembering that tryptophan is carried into the brain via carbohydrate," wrote White, adding "another reason to have your protein and carbs dinner."

Deficiency of serotonin is linked to many negative things, including sleep problems.

Best Time to Eat Dinner

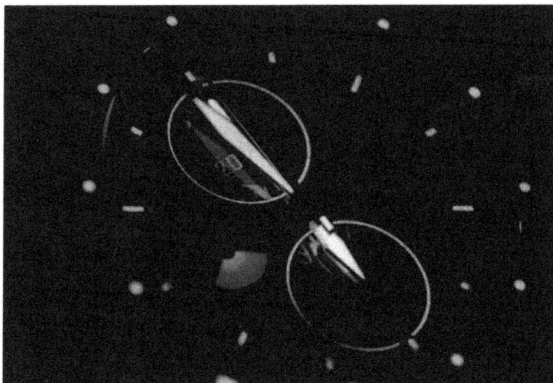

Photo Credit: Eric Kilby.

Dinner, as you know now, is an important meal. Back at lunch we came to the calculation that for this program you would have your lunch around 12:30pm.

At lunch time, we discussed Dr. Oz's 2010 program, in which he teamed up with   Sharecare and the Nike SPARQ Training Network to offer 11-week free program he called *Move It to Lose It*. We discussed how on week 5 there was a video in which Dr. Oz is talking to a woman who woke up early but didn't have her breakfast until 9am, ate her lunch at 1pm, and who had her dinner usually around 6pm.

He told her that in reality she should have had her breakfast at 7:30, or within an hour of waking up, and that she should have had lunch around 12pm and that dinner should be had around 6:30pm.

He said that six-and-half hours after lunch one should

have their dinner, meaning for our program the best time to eat dinner would be around 7pm.

However, what time you eat dinner depends on what time you go to bed.

Jamie A. Koufman, a doctor who specializes in acid reflux wrote for the *New York Times* on the issue. "To stop the remarkable increase in reflux disease, we have to stop eating by 8 p.m., or whatever time falls at least three hours before bed," wrote Koufman.

Now, we need to do some math. Remember that during the early part of this book I told you about a psychologist named Michael J. Breus, who happens to be the author of *Good Night: The Sleep Doctor's 4-Week Program to Better Sleep and Better Health*, who said that everyone can figure out their perfect bedtime by adjusting their preferred wake-up time to the time they go to bed.

Since I encouraged you to wake up at 6am, that means you would want to go to bed at 10:45pm.

If we incorporate Koufman's suggestion of three hours into that, it would mean the best time to have dinner for this program would be around 7:30-7:45.

So, enjoy your dinner at 7:30!

Dinner Recipe

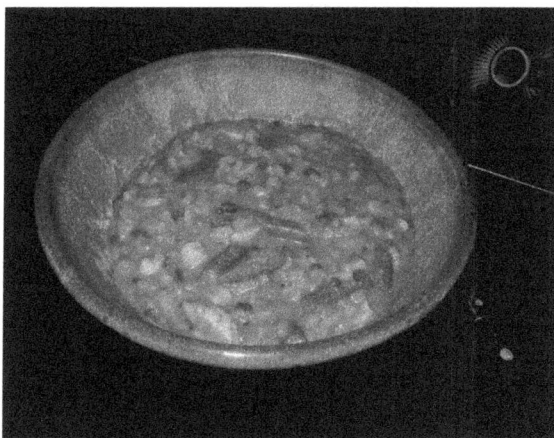

Photo Credit: Tony Alter.

This is the final recipe I'm recommending. Dinner is such an important meal, and, of course, it makes sense to have a healthy dinner.

Lentils are really great! According to *Self* magazine, a cup of lentils, mature seeds, cooked, boiled, without salt contains about 230 calories in a 3% fat, 70% carbohydrate and 27% protein.

"One cup of 'em cooked delivers 16 grams of appetite-curbing fiber and 18 grams of protein," Sarah-Jane Bedwell, a registered dietitian, told *Self*, saying it was a super food. "Lentils also cook up quicker than other legumes and easily absorb the flavors of other dishes," adding that she prefers red lentils to other colors because they cook around 15 minutes and don't need soaking.

Once again, we have a recipe from the USDA's *Healthy Eating on a Budget Cookbook*. This recipe makes 10 servings, and each has about 110 calories, 1g of fat, 20g of carbohydrate, and 6g of protein.

Lentil Stew

Ingredients

2 teaspoons olive oil (or canola oil)

1 onion (large, chopped)

1 teaspoon garlic powder

1 package frozen sliced carrots (16 ounces)

1 package dry lentils (16 ounces, rinsed and drained)

3 cans diced tomatoes (14.5 ounces each)

3 cups water

1 teaspoon chili powder

Directions

1. Heat the oil in a large pot over medium heat.

2. Add chopped onion.

3. Cook for 3 minutes, or until tender.

4. Stir in garlic powder, carrots, lentils, tomatoes, water and chili powder.

5. Simmer, uncovered, for about 20 minutes or until lentils are tender.

The Right Lifestyle

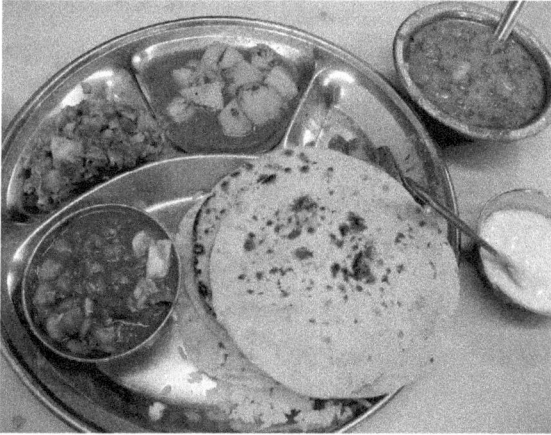

Photo Credit: Yusuke Kawasaki.

Ok, you already know the facts about red and processed meats. Of course, that doesn't mean there isn't any healthy meat.

But let's think about plant-based diets.

What exactly is a plant-based diet? "It is a diet based on fruits, vegetables, tubers, whole grains, and legumes," explain doctors Alona Pulde and Matthew Lederman, the authors of *The Forks Over Knives Plan*, adding that a plant-based diet "excludes or minimizes meat (including chicken and fish), dairy products, and eggs, as well as highly refined foods like bleached flour, refined sugar, and oil."

I think that vegetarian eating gets a bad rap in the United States. People think eating vegetarian meal means it is boring. You see that photo above, taken by Yusuke Kawasaki in India? Does it looking boring to you?

That is thali. It means "plate" in Indian languages like Hindi and Tamil. As such, it is a meal composed of several small meals.

"Most popular meal in India," says the menu at Maya, a restaurant in Poulton-le-Fylde in the UK, adding that it was a "Maharajas all time favourite."

But thali is not healthy.

"Despite its fresh, vegetarian ingredients and home cooked tough," wrote Megan Ogilvie for the Toronto *Star*, adding that one thali they looked at had "just as many calories and as much fat and sodium as a Big Mac combo with large fries and large Coke."

In other words, plant-based diets can also be unhealthy. The idea is not to go extreme from one to the other, but I gave you good ideas in this book for what to eat healthy.

This is about healthy lifestyle, not about dieting. When your lifestyle is healthy, I promise you that you will eat better, too.

My #1 advice for eating right is to download (or print) the USDA's *Healthy Eating on a Budget Cookbook*. You can find it by Googling or going to the usda.gov website and searching in the search box.

What I love about this book is that it gives you cost reference, so you know how much the meals will cost. You also get to know the serving amount, so that you can store it nicely!

This is also a book that is not vegan or even vegetarian, although both can find their space, but a book that gives you an overall wellness focused healthy meals. You will find chicken and fish and tofu and all sorts of diverse stuff.

It is also free!

Make Love Early

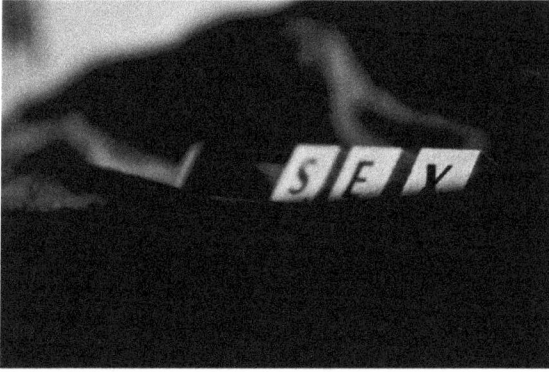

Photo Credit: Sarah Scicluna.

If you have kids, this sounds like a luxury. After dinner, there might be cleaning of the dishes. You might be getting the kids ready for bed. Or you're just too stressed out from it all.

But sex is very important, and we must make the time.

Abraham Maslow's theory of human needs, which we learn about in the beginning of this book, says that sex is important in two places: in physiological needs, where like food and water it was listed as a basic need; and in love and belonging, where with family and friendship it was listed as a mid-level need.

"Sex is an integral component of our social interactions, relationships, and spiritual identities," agrees Jessica O'Reilly, in her book *The New Sex Bible: The New Guide to Sexual Love*.

O'Reilly, who has a doctorate in human sexuality, also writes in her book that physical affection has many benefits such as deepening your bond with your loved one, reducing stress, and even promoting a restful sleep.

Chiara Atik, a journalist who writes for *The Date Report*, says that 8 to 10 pm is the prime time for sex. "Women are totally energized and ready to initiate sex at this time," wrote Atik, who used material from Russia for her article, adding that men are also ready at that time and such "this is the best time of day to have sex."

Types of Sex

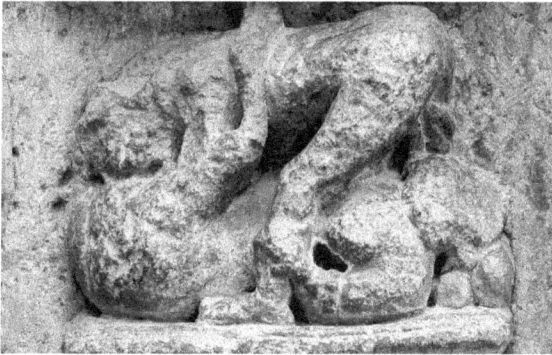

Photo Credit: Nagarjun Kandukuru.

Sex, like anything else in life, comes in different forms.

Debby Herbenick, a sexologist and author of *Because It Feels Good: A Woman's Guide to Sexual Pleasure and Satisfaction*, says that sometimes we want to feel one way and do a sexual act; and then might feel another way and do another sexual act.

"What kind of sex do you want?" Herbenick asks in her book. She then gives a list of words or phrases that best describe how one might like sex to feel and asks the reader to place "m" or "i" in front, the m standing for masturbation while the i stands for intercourse.

These words or phrases, 68 of them divided into four columns, go from being flirtatious to orgasmic.

"Like any journey, the path to pleasurable sex is made easier if you have an idea of where you'd like to go," writes

Herbenick in her book.

For *Men's Health*, Herbenick said that masturbation is great for both sexes. She listed one of the benefits of masturbating before bed as a good way to fall sleep.

Sex, of course, is not just about intercourse or masturbation. Oral sex, for example, has been around since ancient times.

"A well-known French paleontologist by the name of Yves Coppens suggested that the famous Lucy (the first prehistoric woman) practiced a sort of 'paleo-fellatio,'" wrote journalist Annie Auguste for *Salon*.

Then there's anal sex.

Jane Greer, sex therapist and the author of *What About Me? Stop Selfishness From Ruining Your Relationship*, told *Women's Health* magazine editors that the biggest "misconception about anal sex is that it is disgusting, dirty, messy, or that it hurts," adding that "anal sex can be an extremely erotic, exciting activity."

Benefits of Sex

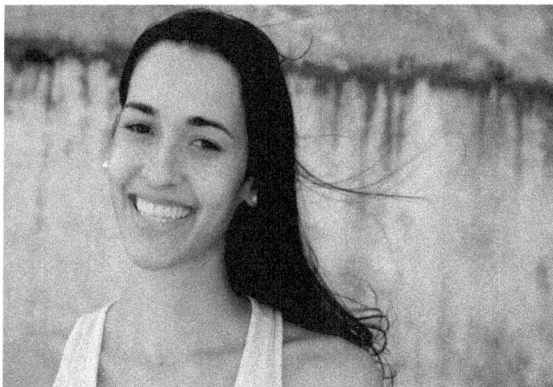

Photo Credit: Marina Aguiar.

There are many benefits to sex. Aside from feeling good, and let's admit it because it does, scientists have long advocated for people understanding its benefits, too.

According to Ray Morgan, a doctor and the author of *Food For Thought: 25 Ways to Protect Yourself from Disease and Promote Excellent Health*, semen is good for you.

"It gives a shot of zinc, calcium, potassium, fructose and proteins; it is a veritable cornucopia of vitality," writes Morgan in the book, also citing a study in which females who had sex without condom showed less signs of depression than ones who had sex with condoms (Morgan has a safe sex caution in the book).

Jon Schiller, author of *Prostate Cancer*, writes in his book about a study in which high frequency of ejaculation in males was related to decreased risk of prostate cancer.

When men orgasm, their prostate is stimulated. As such, the activity seems to help it in use, so to speak.

Being sexually active is also good for women, too. When we age, for example, our vaginas feel it those aging side effects, because our vagina well-being depends on our hormones.

"Vaginal atrophy, also called atrophic vaginitis, is thinning, drying and inflammation of the vaginal walls due to your body having less estrogen," explains *Mayo Clinic*, adding that it occurs often after menopause but that it can also "develop during breast-feeding or at any other time your body's estrogen production declines."

One of the suggested ways to help reduce the chances of getting that nasty condition is by having regular sex.

"While prevention may not be possible, steps can be taken to keep your vaginal tissues healthy," says Bayor College of Medicine's *Obstetrics and Gynecology* website, noting that regular sexy is a good step in the right direction as it "enhances blood flow to your vagina."

In other words, the more action your vagina gets the more blood there is down there, and thus making the vagina more healthy.

Best Time To Have Sex

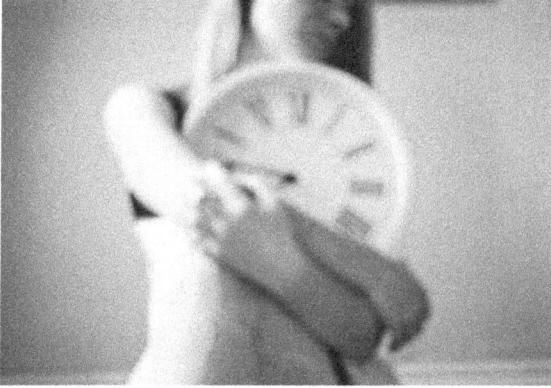

Photo Credit: Lauren Hammond.

No matter what kind of sex you choose, best thing to do is to do it early. However, not too early.

According to top doctors who spoke with *CBS News,* for their "Better Erections: 11 Secrets from Top Doc" story, a man's erection needs a good amount of blood. But so does his stomach after eating, which needs blood to digest the food.

"A full stomach is likely to mess with a woman's sex drive as well," says Dana Dovey, the health and science journalist for *Medical Daily,* adding that it can also make a woman feel bloated and not sexy.

So, how long do you need to wait? Couple of hours.

That means, if you followed this program and had your dinner at 7:30pm, you might want to wait until around 9:30

to try and have your hot sex.

Don't worry; it will still leave you an hour and fifteen minutes of playtime before you're going to bed at 10:45pm.

Enjoy yourself.

Say Thank You

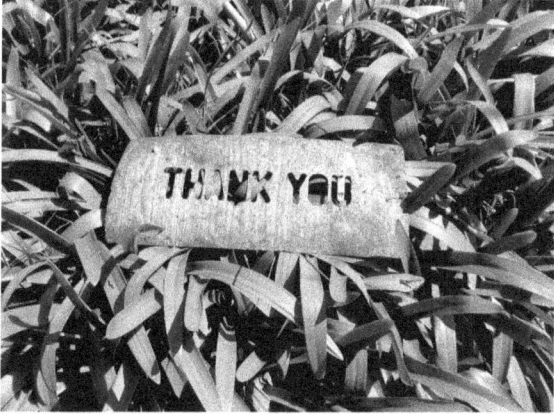

Photo Credit: Kimberly Appelcline.

"If you concentrate on what you have, you will always end up having more, even if it is just 2 dollars," said Oprah Winfrey, to a room full of Canadian guests who came to see her during her Lifeclass Tour. "If you focus on what you don't have, you will never, ever, ever have enough."

Oprah, who says she started the practice of writing 5 things she's grateful for at the end of the day 16 years earlier, said it was the single most important thing she has ever done in her life.

Sarah Ban Breathnach, the author of *Simple Abundance*, whose book remained on the New York Times Best Sellers list for 119 weeks, selling around 7 million copies, introduced Oprah to the concept.

In the book, Ban Breathnach asks her readers to keep a

gratitude journal and write at least five things one is grateful for.

Robert A. Emmons, a professor of psychology at UC Davis, has been studying gratitude for a long time. Emmons, the author of *Thanks!: How Practicing Gratitude Can Make You Happier*, says that gratitude works in two phases: first phase is acknowledging of the goodness in our lives; while the second phase is recognizing that the sources of this gratitude is outside of the self.

"Gratefulness is a knowing awareness that we are the recipients of goodness," writes Emmons in his book. "In gratitude we remember the contributions that others have made for the sake of our well-being."

Amy Morin, a psychotherapist and the author of *13 Things Mentally Strong People Don't Do*, says there are many scientific benefits to gratitude. In her book, she recommends to start small, being grateful for things that you take for granted. For example, she mentions that if you're reading her book you're already in a better position than the one billion people worldwide that cannot read.

In an article for *Forbes* magazine, Morin listed seven scientific benefits of gratitude: that grateful people tend to have more relationships; that physical and mental health are improved by it; that it helps people sleep better; that self esteem is improved by it; and that it increases mental strength.

In other words, gratitude is no longer just some hoopla. It is real. It is real for entrepreneurs like Oprah Winfrey, and it is real for scientists like Robert A. Emmons and Amy Morin.

About Kelly

Kelly Williams is a writer who lives in the United States. The books by the author are based on own personal growth, following sound advice from experts at the top in their field, to live a better life.

For more books from **011 Media**, visit our website:
www.011-media.co